Handling Difficult Situations

Core Principles of Acute Neurology:
Recognizing Brain Injury
Providing Acute Care
Communicating Prognosis

Handling Difficult Situations

EELCO F. M. WIJDICKS, M.D., PH.D., FNCS, FANA

Professor of Neurology, Mayo Clinic College of Medicine

Chair, Division of Critical Care Neurology

Consultant, Neurosciences Intensive Care Unit

Saint Marys Hospital

Mayo Clinic, Rochester, Minnesota

OXFORD
UNIVERSITY PRESS

OXFORD
UNIVERSITY PRESS

Oxford University Press is a department of the University of Oxford.
It furthers the University's objective of excellence in research, scholarship,
and education by publishing worldwide.

Oxford   New York
Auckland   Cape Town   Dar es Salaam   Hong Kong   Karachi
Kuala Lumpur   Madrid   Melbourne   Mexico City   Nairobi
New Delhi   Shanghai   Taipei   Toronto

With offices in
Argentina   Austria   Brazil   Chile   Czech Republic   France   Greece
Guatemala   Hungary   Italy   Japan   Poland   Portugal   Singapore
South Korea   Switzerland   Thailand   Turkey   Ukraine   Vietnam

Oxford is a registered trademark of Oxford University Press
in the UK and certain other countries.

Published in the United States of America by
Oxford University Press
198 Madison Avenue, New York, NY 10016

© 2014 by Mayo Foundation for Medical Education and Research.

Library of Congress Cataloging–in–Publication Data
Wijdicks, Eelco F. M., 1954– author.
Handling difficult situations / Eelco F. M. Wijdicks.
    p. ; cm. — (Core principles of acute neurology)
Includes bibliographical references.
ISBN 978–0–19–992876–7 (alk. paper)
I. Title.   II. Series: Core principles of acute neurology.
[DNLM: 1. Brain Diseases—diagnosis.   2. Brain Diseases—therapy.   3. Acute Disease.
4. Decision Making.   5. Neurologic Manifestations.   6. Neurology—methods. WL 141]
RC355
616.8—dc23
2013033305

The science of medicine is a rapidly changing field. As new research and clinical experience broaden
our knowledge, changes in treatment and drug therapy occur. The author and publisher of this
work have checked with sources believed to be reliable in their efforts to provide information that
is accurate and complete, and in accordance with the standards accepted at the time of publication.
However, in light of the possibility of human error or changes in the practice of medicine, neither
the author, nor the publisher, nor any other party who has been involved in the preparation or
publication of this work warrants that the information contained herein is in every respect accurate
or complete. Readers are encouraged to confirm the information contained herein with other
reliable sources, and are strongly advised to check the product information sheet provided by the
pharmaceutical company for each drug they plan to administer.

9 8 7 6 5 4 3 2 1
Printed in the United States of America
on acid-free paper

For Barbara, Coen, and Marilou

Contents

Preface

Handling acute neurologic conditions is an out-and-out challenge for most physicians. Decision-making in acute neurologic conditions is tough, as there is a cornucopia of judgments to make in caring for an unstable disorder. Nonetheless, in many acute neurologic disorders there is good appreciation of how to approach the patient.

Skilled specialized physicians have a repertoire of clinical signs and findings that warn them of trouble ahead. From the viewpoint of everyone else there are many unexpected situations. There are clinical scenarios that continue to come up and always generate questions on management. When is coma reversible and what are the causes that should be recognized? What is the next step in seizure control? How can we asses the severity of acute spinal cord injury? How can we best manage acute stroke with endovascular options available? How do we assess life-threatening neuromuscular disorders? When do we urgently consult a neurosurgeon? What could we do differently in transplant recipients? How do we avoid errors on a CT scan?

This book discusses these pressing questions facing neurologists and, frankly, any physician. These are questions that are always approached with a sense of insecurity but that require answers to appropriately care for the patient. In so doing a separate volume is useful but only if it provides straightforward information and advice. These are often split-second decision and this volume provides common examples on how to deal with it.

Introduction to the Series

The confrontation with an acutely ill neurologic patient is quite an unsettling situation for physicians, but all will have to master how to manage the patient at presentation, how to shepherd the unstable patient to an intensive care unit, and how to take charge. To do that aptly, knowledge of the principles of management is needed. Books on the clinical practice of acute, emergency, and critical care neurology have appeared, but none have yet treated the fundamentals in depth.

Core Principles of Acute Neurology is a series of short volumes that handles topics not found in sufficient detail elsewhere. The books focus precisely on those areas that require a good working knowledge. These are: the consequences of acute neurologic diseases, medical care in all its aspects and relatedness with the injured brain, difficult decisions in complex situations. Because the practice involves devastatingly injured patients, there is a separate volume on prognostication and neuropalliation. Other volumes are planned in the future.

The series has unique features. I hope to contextualize basic science with clinical practice in a readable narrative with a light touch and without wielding the jargon of this field. The ten chapters in each volume try to spell out in the clearest terms how things work. The text is divided into a description of principles followed by its relevance to practice— keeping it to the bare essentials. There are boxes inserted into the text with quick reminders ("By the Way") and useful percentages carefully researched and vetted for accuracy ("By the Numbers"). Drawings are used to illustrate mechanisms and pathophysiology.

These books cannot cover an entire field, but brevity and economy allows a focus on one topic at a time. Gone are the days of large, doorstop tomes with many words on paper but with little practical value. This series is therefore characterized by simplicity—in a good sense—and it is acute and critical care neurology at the core, not encyclopedic but representative. I hope it supplements clinical curricula or comprehensive textbooks.

The audience is primarily neurologists and neurointensivists, neurosurgeons, fellows, and residents. Neurointensivists have increased in numbers, and many major institutions have attendings and fellowship programs. However, these books cross disciplines and should also be useful for intensivists, anesthesiologists, emergency physicians, nursing staff, and allied health care professionals in intensive care units and the emergency department. In the end the intent is to write a book that provides a sound reassuring basis to practice well, and that helps with understanding and appreciating the complexities of care of a patient with an acute neurologic condition.

1

Treatable Coma

If a patient becomes comatose and stays comatose, the common presumption is that there is a major and permanent brain injury. Depending on where the patient is seen first, different scenarios come into play. The "top three" causes of coma are therefore variable. On the street and in the field, intoxication or illicit drug use, diabetic dysregulation, and environmental causes are considered most likely.[5,17] When patients are first encountered in the emergency department, traumatic brain injury (often accompanied by alcohol intoxication), anoxic-ischemic brain injury after cardiac arrest, and drug overdose or poisoning remain the most common causes of coma, especially among young adults.[6] Intoxications include ethanol, heroin, and sedative-hypnotics or a less distinctive street pill. The distribution of causes of coma is different in patients seen in the hospital or intensive care units—structural causes of brain injury are then more frequent.

Given that we can do only so much in acute coma, keeping a treatable cause of coma from going awry should be a priority. Treatable coma can be defined as coma that can be reversed by a specific action by the attending physician. It is important to be aware that there are immediate actions that could lead to awakening of the patient, and actions that lead to avoidance of the secondary effects of the acute brain lesion. For many patients, a complex medical or neurosurgical intervention or combination of both would be indicated.

When a physician has to evaluate a suddenly unresponsive patient, the first questions should always be: How do I rapidly diagnose the cause, and what test do I look at first? What can the general examination say about the potential of an intoxication being the cause? When is a presentation out of the ordinary? How can I reverse this condition? Common misjudgments include failure to recognize the need for correction of a new metabolic abnormality, to fail to appreciate the availability of specific antidotes and dialysis, to wait with treatments for brain swelling, and to delay beneficial effects of an acute neurosurgical intervention.

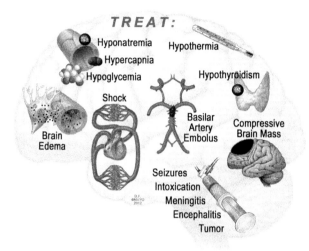

Figure 1.1 Acute interventions to consider in coma.

Principles

The interventions that potentially reverse coma are shown in Figure 1.1. There is an understandable urgency to avoid long-term effects. Each of these causes are further explored here.

CLASSIFICATION OF COMA

Before we consider treatable causes of coma, we should revisit the five major categories of coma.[28] The division of coma into separate categories remains one of the more standard principles and is clinically useful because it focuses the physician on systematically working through major causes of coma. Combinations are possible but uncommon. Coma from severe alcohol intoxication may result in a fatal traumatic brain injury, but in many other instances, one overriding cause can be singled out (Table 1.1).

There are several important principles when structural brain injury is concerned. Cortical activation resulting in awareness and alertness requires several active structures. These are the thalamus, basal forebrain, posterior hypothalamus, and brainstem nuclei in the ascending reticular activating system. A mass may compress, displace, or destroy these structures.[27] A unilateral hemispheric lesion without pressure on the opposite hemisphere will not decrease level of consciousness because, traditionally, bilateral lesions are needed to interrupt the thalamocortical connections. Bilateral hemispheric lesions impair the function of the thalamus by interrupting the thalamocortical circuitry and frontoparietal connections that are essential in maintaining alertness.[8] Acute expanding lesions in the cerebellum may compress the dorsal brainstem and thus the ascending reticular activating system.

Table 1.1 **Categorization of Coma**

Structural Brain Injury
Hemisphere with mass effect
Bilateral hemispheres
Cerebellum with mass effect
Brainstem

Acute Metabolic-Endocrine Derangement
Sodium abnormalities
Glucose abnormalities
Liver failure
Renal failure
Hypercapnia
Hyperammonemia
Hypothyroidism

Diffuse Physiologic Brain Dysfunction
Seizures
Poisoning
Drug use
Hypothermia

Psychogenic Unresponsiveness
Acute catatonia
Conversion disorder

When it comes down to diffuse dysfunction of the brain, many acute metabolic or endocrine derangements may lead to neuronal depression. These abnormalities are usually quickly reversible. Reversal may lead to dramatic improvement of patient responsiveness. Acute metabolic derangement will result in deepening coma if not treated promptly. One should keep them in mind and order appropriate laboratory tests. These derangements cause neuronal hypometabolism, but some lead to structural brain injuries. (For example, acute hyperglycemia may result in brain edema that cannot be easily reversed.) Moreover, anoxic-ischemic injury may occur when marked hypoxemia or shock accompanies a severe acute metabolic derangement. Endocrine crises such as hypoglycemia or hyperglycemia, thyroid coma, or panhypopituitarism all may have specific brain lesions, but are much less defined and usually reversible. Similar situations occur in patients with fulminant hepatic failure that leads to cerebral edema. Likewise, improvement after recovery of multiorgan failure is expected, but there may be neurologic sequelae as a result of shock and hypoxemia.

Rarely observed is psychiatric unresponsiveness, which may include dramatic and potentially lethal disorders such as acute catatonia or neuroleptic malignant syndrome. Usually these manifestations occur in a patient with an established psychiatric disorder.

Once aware of these mechanisms and neurologic findings, the next core principle is to localize the lesion using key elements of the neurologic examination.[26] Localization starts with the conceptual division of the brain into hemispheres and brainstem. The tentorium is also often used as a dividing anatomical structure—lesions above and below the tentorium refer to the hemispheres versus brainstem and cerebellum. Coma can be caused by a bihemispheric syndrome or a brainstem syndrome. Brainstem syndrome can be further divided into intrinsic brainstem syndrome or brainstem displacement syndrome.[27]

Bihemispheric syndrome is characterized by the common absence of any specific localizing findings. Patients may have a gaze preference; the brainstem reflexes are intact; pupils may be small or normal; motor responses are usually withdrawal to pain, extensor responses, or none. Localization to a noxious stimulus may occur if patients are more "to the surface" or recovering from coma. In some patients, myoclonus or focal twitches can be seen. The breathing patterns can be periodic but are usually regular. Nothing points to a specific area in the brain hemispheres—hence the term—and lesions may be in the cortex, white matter, or thalamus.

Brainstem syndromes can be divided into intrinsic brainstem syndromes and brainstem displacement syndromes. These two syndromes may overlap in a clinical sense. An intrinsic brainstem syndrome (due to primary lesion inside the brainstem) is characterized by extensor posturing or flexion of the motor response, skew deviation, miosis or anisocoria, and often abnormal oculovestibular responses. With 50 cc ice water injection into the ear, an internuclear ophthalmoplegia can be brought to bear. The eye on the same side as the injected ear moves toward the ear, while there is failure to move the eye that is opposite to the injected ear. The finding of internuclear ophthalmoplegia is specific for a lesion of the medial longitudinal fasciculus that courses through the brainstem connecting the III and VI cranial nerve nuclei—it is a useful sign of an acute lesion in the brainstem.

Brainstem displacement syndromes (due to a mass moving the brainstem laterally) can be above or below the tentorium. Above the tentorium, hemispheric lesions compress the thalamus and mesencephalon. In these patients, a unilateral fixed and dilated (varying from 5 to 7 mm) pupil is seen and, if untreated, is usually followed by bilateral fixed mid-position pupils. The fixed and dilated pupil is a result of a stretch injury to the oculomotor nerve or damage to its nucleus due to ischemia from displacement of the brainstem vasculature. The pontine reflexes are intact initially, but may disappear if the syndrome progresses.

Brainstem displacement syndrome can be due to a lesion centrally located within the brain above the tentorium that compresses the thalamus, causing a vertical downward torque that buckles the mesencephalon. Early fixed mid-position

Table 1.2 **Anatomy of Coma and Key Clinical Features**

Location	Clinical Pointers
Bihemispheric	Spontaneous eye movements (roving, dipping, ping-pong)
	Upward or downward eye deviation
	Intact oculovestibular responses
	Intact pupil and corneal reflexes
	Variable motor responses
	Myoclonus
Intrinsic Brainstem	Skew deviation
	Internuclear ophthalmoplegia
	Vertical nystagmus or bobbing
	Miosis
	Variable pupil or corneal reflexes (may both be absent)
	Absent oculocephalic or oculovestibular responses
	Extensor or flexion motor responses
Brainstem displacement	Anisocoria or unilateral fixed wide pupil
(from hemispheric or	(lateral displacement from hemispheric mass)
cerebellar mass)	Mid-position fixed pupils
	(downward central displacement from hemispheric mass)
	Absent corneal reflexes and intact pupil reflexes
	(displacement from cerebellar mass)
	Extensor or withdrawal motor responses

pupils from mesencephalic interruption are seen with variable motor responses; and in general, pontine reflexes remain intact.

Brainstem displacement below the tentorium is usually from a lesion in the cerebellum. In those patients, bilateral miosis and loss of both corneal reflexes and oculocephalic reflexes from pontine compression are far more predominant and found early in the clinical course.[24] The main findings of these syndromes are summarized in Table 1.2.

The next core principle is to link the CT scan abnormalities to the clinical findings. Discrepancies between a CT scan lesion and clinical findings may indicate the lesion has progressed since the first CT. Such a discrepancy may also be caused by additional new laboratory abnormalities that can further reduce the level of consciousness, or by recent administration of a central nervous system (CNS) depressant drug.[10]

A final principle is that a brain lesion may cause deterioration from secondary swelling that may displace the brainstem, causing permanent brainstem injury. This initial injury may be quickly defining, and little can be done if the brainstem reflexes disappear in a caudal direction. This sequence is commonly fixed pupils (mesencephalon) followed by absent corneal reflexes, followed by absent oculocephalic responses (pons) and absent cough response, followed by apnea and hypotension due to loss of vascular tone (medulla oblongata). A large hemispheric mass may progress in such a direction.

In Practice

The primary focus in management of a comatose patient remains—as in any unstable patient—correction of abnormal vital signs and subsequent immediate correction of laboratory abnormalities.[28] The first priority is to assess for adequate oxygenation and to improve oxygenation, which may simply require a nasal cannula. Oxygen delivered by nasal prongs may provide an FiO_2 of 40% at 5–6 L/min, but a face mask with 10-L oxygen flow may be needed to maintain a pulse oximeter reading of more than 95%.

The degree of coma does not necessarily dictate the need for intubation but the airway needs to be secured. Therefore, the mnemonic "GCS of 8, intubate" is not only nondescriptive, it is incomplete and perhaps inaccurate. It is prudent to intubate any comatose patient with irregular ineffective breathing drive and poor oxygenation. A comatose patient with a major facial injury most often needs emergency tracheostomy. The patient may need to be intubated if there is airway obstruction (important clinical cues are increased work of breathing, pooling secretions, or even gurgling sounds). The patient will need to be reintubated if a laryngeal tube has been placed in the field.

At the same time, one may have to correct hypotension by placing the patient in Trendelenburg position and adding crystalloids (rapid bolus infusion of 500 cc normal saline followed by additional bolus if needed) and, if no response, to start vasopressors (phenylephrine bolus up to 200 mcg). If hypotension is caused by a major cardiac arrhythmia, more specific treatment is needed, often including ventricular rate control. In a hypertensive patient, it is important to correct extreme hypertension with intravenous labetalol, hydralazine, or nicardipine (all three antihypertensives can start with a 10 mg IV dose). Systolic blood pressure above 200 mm Hg or mean arterial blood pressure above 120 mm Hg are urgent triggers for intervention.

It is important to treat temperature abnormalities and to correct hypothermia with warming blankets or, conversely, hyperthermia with cooling blankets and icepacks.

The next step is to look at the laboratory values that should have come back by now. However, no harm is done if a patient with a high likelihood of hypoglycemia is given 50 mL/50% glucose solution with co-administration of 100 mg thiamine IV even before the blood sugar is known. Treatment of severe hyponatremia (less than 120 mmol/L) involves hypertonic saline (3% hypertonic saline, 100 cc/h).

Treatment of hypercalcemia is by saline rehydration infusion followed by parenteral bisphosphonate pamidronate.

When toxins are suspected, antidotes can be considered. One may administer naloxone (0.4 to 2 mg every 3 minutes IV) if opioid use is strongly suspected, or flumazenil (slow IV administration at 0.2 mg per minute up to 1 mg), if benzodiazepine toxicity is suspected. However, as it may provoke seizures, flumazenil is contraindicated in patients with a seizure disorder and in whom concomitant tricyclic antidepressant overdose is suspected. Flumazenil may bring on seizures associated with tricyclic antidepressant overdose. Under these circumstances, one should consider administration of charcoal or elimination of the toxin by hemodialysis or hemoperfusion—or simply ICU support until the drug washes out.

Now being familiar with the principles of initial management of the comatose patient, a cause should be found. This requires three pieces of information: (1) a specific history from family members, paramedics, or bystanders; (2) a detailed neurologic examination tailored toward the clinical condition; and (3) a recent CT scan of the brain. The next questions that the examiner will have to ask are whether coma is due to destructive structural brain lesion or to a global acute physiological derangement of brain function. If there is a structural lesion, where is it located—in both the cerebral hemispheres or in the brainstem?

First, the history should focus on whether coma is due to intoxication. Were there pills or over-the-counter drugs or herbs that the patient had access to? Has the patient had a psychiatric consultation or admission and made a prior suicide attempt? Is there a prior history of drug or drinking habits?

The next questions should focus on the possibility of a CNS infection. Did the patient use antibiotics to treat infection, and was there rapid onset of fever and headache? Was the patient confused while there was fever, and were there difficulties getting the words out?

The possibility of diabetes should also be taken into account. Did the patient have prior episodes of diabetic ketoacidosis, and has there been a change in diabetic medication? Could the patient have overdosed on hypoglycemic drugs? If the patient is not diabetic, is anyone in the family a diabetic using medication that the patient could have taken?

Finally, could the patient be in nonconvulsive status epilepticus or in a postictal state, and have there been prior seizures or is the patient a known epileptic? These questions are very pertinent, particularly if the initial CT scan is completely normal.

All of this information is obtained while examining the patient or even before tests are ordered. A detailed medical and neurologic examination follows. Neurologic examination can determine the cause and severity of coma, but there might also be clues from a general physical examination that may point toward a certain cause. The examination of the pupils is important and may reveal important findings. Small or pinpoint pupils (<2 mm) can be due to a pontine lesion but, more often, are due to opioid (e.g., heroin or atypical antipsychotics) overdose. Midsize light-fixed pupils are due to a midbrain lesion and always indicate more severe injury and loss of brainstem function.[3] Maximally dilated pupils (>8 mm) are due to a lesion of the third cranial nerve nuclei in the mesencephalon or compression of the peripheral fibers. In a comatose patient a unilateral fixed pupil is due to a third cranial nerve lesion from compression of the midbrain, retraction of the third nerve, or pressure of the nerve against the clivus due to mass effect. Again, drugs and toxins dilate the pupils, and known examples are cocaine and amphetamines.

Eye movement abnormalities have less localizing value. However, many spontaneous eye movement abnormalities do indicate a structural lesion. These are ping-pong (rapid horizontal movements every few seconds) and ocular dipping (slow downward and rapid upward movements of both eyes). An important finding is that spontaneous roving eye movements indicate that the brainstem is intact. On the other hand, skew deviation of the eyes suggests an acute brainstem injury. Any forced deviation of the eyes to one side indicates an ipsilateral hemispheric or a contralateral pontine lesion. Forced eye gaze may also be a sign of ongoing seizures and can be seen in partial complex seizures or nonconvulsive status epilepticus.

Motor responses in comatose patients clearly indicate the severity of bihemispheric or brainstem damage and may change with deepening of coma. These motor responses point toward the likelihood of a structural lesion in both cerebral hemispheres or in the brainstem, and typically evolve during worsening.

Myoclonus, asterixis, and seizures (partial or generalized) may be observed relatively early and during progression of symptoms. Myoclonus can be generalized or multifocal and typically occurs after an extensive anoxic-ischemic injury but can be associated with certain drugs (e.g. lithium). This asynchronic twitching of multiple muscle groups may include face and trunk.

While examining the patient it is important to consider a toxidrome.[21] There may be useful cues. First, profuse sweating, bronchorrhea, salivation and miosis may indicate a poisoning with cholinergic agents, insecticides, and weaponized nerve gas. Dryness of skin indicates barbiturate poisoning or anticholinergic agents such as antiparkinson drugs, antipsychotics, antispasmotics and tricyclic antidepressants. A serotonin syndrome may present with mydriasis and myoclonus and often these patients have marked rigidity. Hypotension may indicate overdose with antihypertensives.[5,27]

The core temperature is extremely valuable information and is not always known. Fever is another important sign and opens up a large differential diagnosis. In comatose patients, fever is presumed due to a CNS infection until excluded or found to be due to another source. Hypothermia is typically the result of an alcohol intoxication, an overdose of barbiturates, or an overdose of tricyclic depressants. Hyperthermia can be seen with cocaine, tricyclic antidepressants and salicylate intoxication.

Table 1.3 **Thresholds of Laboratory Values Compatible with Altered Consciousness**

Derangement	Serum
Hyponatremia	<110 mmol/L
Hypernatremia	>160 mmol/L
Hypercalcemia	>15 mg/dL
Hypermagnesemia	>5 mg/dL
Hypercapnia	>70 mm Hg
Hypoglycemia	<40 mg/dL
Hyperglycemia	>600 mg/L

The classic foul breaths should be known and are occasionally helpful.

- Urinary odor: uremia
- Sweat odor: ketoacidosis
- Fish odor: acute hepatic failure
- Garlic odor: organophosphates

Several laboratory tests are immediately relevant. These are glucose, hematocrit, full blood count, platelet count and blood smear, electrolytes, glucose, blood urea nitrogen, creatinine, liver function tests, osmolality, serum ammonia, and arterial blood gas. A significant change must have occurred or passed a certain threshold. These values are shown in Table 1.3.

Thyroid function should be measured if myxedema coma is considered. In any patient with an intoxication, urine screening and blood screening are needed. Blood cultures are needed in any patient with fever and suspicion of CNS infection. If the patient has metabolic acidosis, it is important to identify an anion gap, which is seen with methanol, ethanol, or salicylate intoxication (Table 1.4).[11,21] The anion gap can be calculated from the serum electrolytes. The anion gap = [Na+] – [Cl–] – [HCO3–]. Increase of the anion gap occurs because there is an additional anion, usually lactate from poor tissue perfusion. A gap of 5–15 mEq/L is normal. Ketones with a marked anion gap in metabolic acidosis suggest diabetes-induced ketoacidosis or salicylate poisoning. The absence of ketones in a patient with a marked anion gap indicates atypical alcohols.

An osmolar gap can be calculated to determine accumulation of osmotically active solute. This is particularly important with atypical alcohols such as methanol, ethylene glycol, and isopropyl glycol because they all increase the osmolar gap. The osmolar gap is calculated using the equation $2 \times [Na] + glucose/18 + BUN/2.8$. Calculated osmolality is less than the measured osmolarity and should be no more than 10 mOsm/L.

Table 1.4 **Blood Gas Abnormalities due to Toxins**

Metabolic Acidosis	Respiratory Acidosis
Methanol	Barbiturates
Ethanol	Benzodiazepines
	Opioids
Isoniazid	Strychnine
Salicylates	Tetrodotoxin
Metabolic Alkalosis	*Respiratory Alkalosis*
Diuretics	Salicylates
Nonketotic hyperglycemia	Amphetamines
Lithium	Anticholinergics
	Cocaine
	Cyanide

The CT scan is usually normal in a treatable cause of coma. Many critical situations, including carbon monoxide poisoning, asphyxia after cardiopulmonary resuscitation, and acute evolving encephalitis, are associated with normal initial CT scan findings. The CT scan is often also normal in acute basilar artery occlusion, but in retrospect often a hyperdense basilar artery can be identified (Chapter 10). One of the most common errors is failure to identify a hyperdense basilar artery sign in a patient found suddenly comatose. Unfortunately, failure to recognize this abnormality results in a very poor outcome and lost opportunity for endovascular retrieval of the clot.

An MRI scan becomes exceedingly important in the workup of a patient who might have a treatable cause. MRI is often indicated if the cause is unresolved. MR angiogram could show arterial occlusions.[14] MR venogram could show cerebral venous thrombosis, but signal changes should be found in key locations that explain coma. MRI may demonstrate posterior reversible encephalopathy syndrome not clearly imaged on CT scan and any of the more severe leukoencephalopathies associated with illicit drug use.

Electroencephalography (EEG) is of marginal value in acute coma. The detection rate of seizures not obvious by history or examination is less than 10%. More problematic is that the EEG may suggest a toxic encephalopathy while there is an ongoing structural lesion. Obviously status epilepticus or seizures require immediate intervention. The diagnosis and treatment can be assisted by EEG and requires aggressive management with lorazepam, fosphenytoin, or third-line anesthetic drugs.

The first treatment options are shown in Table 1.5. Treatable coma, however, can be due to mass effect and its remote effect or edema that may displace the brainstem, in which case coma can reverse after neurosurgical intervention.

Table 1.5 **Core Principles of Management of Acute Structural Brain Lesions Causing Coma**

- Protect airway, may need to intubate patient
- Correct hypoxemia with nasal catheter, face mask, or nonrebreather
- Elevate the head to 30 degrees (when increased ICP anticipated)
- Flat body position in shock and suspicion of acute basilar artery occlusion
- Mannitol 20% 1 g/kg IV with mass on CT scan
- Hypertonic saline (7%, 10%, or 23% through central venous catheter)
- Ventriculotomy with acute hydrocephalus
- Surgical evacuation of mass lesion
- Dexamethasone (100 mg IV) in tumors
- Dexamethasone 10 mg IV Q4H for bacterial meningitis
- Full antibiotic coverage (ceftriaxone 2g IV Q12H, vancomycin 20 mg/kg Q12H, ampicillin 2 g 4QH) (if applicable)
- Full antiviral coverage (acyclovir 10 mg/kg Q8H) (if applicable)
- Correct coagulopathy (if applicable)

Removal of a mass causing midline shift will reduce the probability of permanent brainstem injury. This approach is needed in traumatic contusions, large lobar hematomas, and gliomas with surrounding edema.[22,25] In patients who have enlarged ventricles, ventriculostomy placement is urgent. Patients may rapidly deteriorate from enlargement of the ventricles, which causes compression and rapid displacement of the brainstem resulting in rapidly deepening coma. Acute obstructive hydrocephalus is commonly caused by an aneurysmal subarachnoid hemorrhage, bacterial meningitis, intraventricular hemorrhage and can be seen in patients with acute aqueductal stenosis, interventricular tumors, pineal tumors, cerebellar mass from tumor or stroke, or an acute shunt malfunction. After a ventriculostomy is placed, the obstructive lesion can be removed. A ventriculostomy is usually placed at 5 mm Hg, but lower levels may be needed to provide adequate cerebrospinal fluid diversion.

An often important first clinical decision is to reduce intracranial pressure. Patients should receive 20% mannitol, usually in a bolus of 1 g/kg, followed by a maintenance dose of 0.25 to 0.75 g/kg every 4 hours. With this treatment, the serum osmolality should be kept around 300 mOsm/kg; and isotonic fluid intake might be necessary to keep the patient normovolemic. Hypertonic saline used in 3%, 10% or 23% solution can be administered but does require a central catheter placement, and therefore in the hyperacute setting is much less practical. Hyperventilation remains important in reducing increased intracranial pressure, aiming at an arterial pCO_2 between 30 and 35 mm Hg. Corticosteroids can also be very useful in reducing intracranial pressure, particularly in patients with a glioma and mass effect. Typically dexamethasone is administered: 10 mg bolus followed by 4 g/IV every 6 hours.

In some patients, a decompressive craniectomy alone, without tissue removal, is sufficient.[16,19] The conditions in which this is most relevant are in patients with cerebral or cerebellar infarcts with rapid swelling or patients with massive traumatic head injury, in particular after a penetrating injury. Removal of a large part of the skull will allow expansion of the brain and will reduce the possibility of permanent brainstem injury from shift or compression.

Not recognizing an infection as the cause of a treatable coma is probably the most consequential error; therefore, a cerebrospinal fluid examination is warranted in most comatose patients with an initial normal CT scan and no other immediate explanation. Moreover, patients can be inadequately treated for bacterial meningitis using inappropriate antibiotics or inappropriate doses. Cefriaxone is often underdosed and should be 2 g IV every 12 hours. The trough goal for vancomycin is measured after the fourth dose to allow for a steady state and is started with 20 mg/kg IV every 12 hours. Ampicillin is often added in patients over 50 years of age.

Herpes simplex encephalitis is typically recognized by an early temporal lobe hypodensity, but MRI scan usually shows abnormal signal intensity in the temporal lobe, orbital frontal, and subinsular regions. Any patient who presents with focal signs (often aphasia) and fever progressing to a decreased level of consciousness should be considered an untreated herpes simplex encephalitis, and these patients should be treated with acyclovir 10 mg/kg initially with adjustment to creatinine clearance while awaiting the result of the CSF-PCR. Opportunistic infections causing coma can be seen in transplant recipients, and most infections are due to *Listeria, Nocardia asteroides, Aspergillus fumigatus, Cryptococcus neoformans*, or *Toxoplasma gondii*, each with specific therapies.

One should recognize that acute uremia, acute thyroid disease, sepsis, hypoglycemia, hyperglycemia, hyponatremia, hypernatremia, acute hypercalcemic crisis, acute hyperammonemia, and severe hypercapnia are disorders that may reduce the level of consciousness and that all are treatable.[18] With the current point-of-care devices, hypoglycemia is often commonly excluded and patients are typically acutely treated. Most patients with hypoglycemia awaken rapidly after 50 mL of D5W (5% dextrose in water). It is often already administered by emergency medical services before patients reach the hospital, in particular if diabetes is known. No awakening indicates a lengthy and deep hypoglycemia and could point toward prolonged unconsciousness.

Acute overdose remains a common presenting complaint in emergency departments (ED).[7,10,13,20,23] There are specific antidotes available (Table 1.6).[2,5] The use of a "coma cocktail" in assessing and managing coma of undetermined cause has not met many proponents.[1,13] Usually, this cocktail consists of a combination of hypertonic dextrose, thiamine hydrochloride, naloxone hydrochloride, and, flumazenil. Its use must be discouraged simply because of the

Table 1.6 **Specific Treatments to Reverse Coma**

Drug	Treatment
Barbiturates	Forced alkaline diuresis, using 50 mEq of NaHCO3, 1 mEq/mL. hemodialysis, vasopressors to treat shock
Tricyclic antidepressants	Forced alkaline diuresis, antiepileptic drugs
Benzodiazepines	Flumazenil IV or support only
Cocaine	Hypothermia, adrenergic blocking or IV lidocaine to treat ventricular tachycardia
Opiates	Naloxone (0.4–2.0 mg every 1 minute)
Acetaminophen	N-acetylcysteine
Ethylene glycol	Fomepizole

possible side effects of naloxone and flumazenil. Naloxone has great efficacy but also potentially serious side effects, such as aspiration from rapid arousal and development of a florid withdrawal syndrome characterized by agitation, diaphoresis, hypertension, dysrhythmias, and pulmonary edema. In addition, after 30 minutes, the patient may again lapse into coma, which if unwitnessed may cause significant respiratory depression and respiratory arrest. A more prudent approach is to prophylactically intubate the patient and to gradually reverse the opiate overdose by administering naloxone, 0.4–2 mg IV, with incremental doubling of doses every 3 minutes.[11] At the first sign of relapse, 0.4–4 mg of naloxone can be given IV or an infusion of 0.8 mg/kg hourly can be initiated.

Flumazenil reverses the effect of any benzodiazepine but has the same major disadvantages as naloxone: rapid arousal and risk of aspiration pneumonitis. In addition, when high doses of flumazenil are administered, seizures may occur. Again, flumazenil is contraindicated in patients with a seizure disorder and in patients in whom concomitant tricyclic antidepressant intoxication is suspected.[9] The recommended dose of flumazenil, by slow IV administration, is 0.2 mg/min up to a total dose of 1 mg.[8] Benzodiazepine overdose, in general, is not life threatening and can be managed with supportive care only.

Coma from alcohol overdose is common in emergency departments, and neurologists are rarely consulted.[20] Fatality may occur from extreme quantities, which is far more common than appreciated. Seizures may occur from binge drinking and can be due to severe hyponatremia or hypoglycemia as well as traumatic brain injury from aggressive behavior or falls. Toxic blood alcohols levels are usually more than 0.20 and always associated with a large osmolar gap. Treatment of recurrent seizures is indicated, and all patients need intensive care unit support with early intubation to avoid aspiration from vomiting next to liberal fluids and intravenous thiamine or a "banana bag" (multivitamins).

Supportive care is also the only option for benzodiazepines and tricyclic antidepressants, although the cardiac manifestations may focus all attention. A temporary pacemaker may be needed in these patients due to bradyarrhythmias and, often characteristic, widened QRS interval.

By the Way

- Many causes of coma are treatable or resolve spontaneously
- Alcohol and drug intoxication are common in the ED
- Anoxic-ischemic encephalopathy is most common in ICU
- Accumulated drug effects are most common in surgical ICU
- Posterior reversible encephalopathy syndrome is common in medical ICU

Treatable Coma by the Numbers

- ~90% of hypoglycemic coma is rapidly reversible using IV glucose
- ~80% of coma due to mass effect is reversible with evacuation
- ~60% of coma after CPR resolves after therapeutic hypothermia
- ~50% of coma and acute hydrocephalus is reversible with ventriculostomy
- ~10% of coma improves with antidotes

Putting It All Together

- Determine location of lesion and mechanism by dividing causes of coma into structural lesion or physiologic neuronal depression
- Link clinical findings with the CT scan and narrow causes
- Look for a toxidrome if the CT scan is normal
- Determine a possible anion gap and osmolar gap
- Administer a specific antidote, not a "cocktail"

References

1. Betten DP, Vohra RB, Cook MD, Matteucci MJ, Clark RF. Antidote use in the critically ill poisoned patient. *J Intensive Care Med* 2006;21:255–277.
2. Brent J, McMartin K, Phillips S, et al. Fomepizole for the treatment of methanol poisoning. *N Engl J Med* 2001;344:424–429.
3. Burns JD, Schiefer TK, Wijdicks EFM. Large and small: a telltale sign of acute pontomesencephalic injury. *Neurology* 2009;72:1707.
4. Edlow JA, Rabinstein AA, Traub SJ, Wijdicks EFM. Diagnosing reversible causes of coma. *Lancet* 2014; in press.
5. Flomenbaum NE, Goldfrank LR, Hoffman R, et al. *Goldfrank's Toxicologic Emergencies* 8th ed. New York, McGraw-Hill Professional, 2006.
6. Forsberg S, Höjer J, Enander C, Ludwigs U. Coma and impaired consciousness in the emergency room: characteristics of poisoning versus other causes. *Emerg Med J* 2009;26:100–102.
7. Gawin FH, Ellinwood EH Jr. Cocaine and other stimulants: actions, abuse, and treatment. *N Engl J Med* 1988;318:1173–1182.
8. Giannopoulos S, Kostadima V, Selvi A, Nicolopoulos P, Kyritsis AP. Bilateral paramedian thalamic infarcts. *Arch Neurol* 2006;63:1652.
9. Gueye PN, Hoffman JR, Taboulet P, Vicaut E, Baud FJ. Empiric use of flumazenil in comatose patients: limited applicability of criteria to define low risk. *Ann Emerg Med* 1996;27:730–735.
10. Henderson A, Wright M, Pond SM. Experience with 732 acute overdose patients admitted to an intensive care unit over six years. *Med J Aust* 1993;158:28–30.
11. Hill JB. Salicylate intoxication. *N Engl J Med* 1973;288:1110–1113.
12. Hoffman JR, Schriger DL, Luo JS. The empiric use of naloxone in patients with altered mental status: a reappraisal. *Ann Emerg Med* 1991;20:246–252.
13. Hoffman RS, Goldfrank LR. The poisoned patient with altered consciousness: controversies in the use of a "coma cocktail." *JAMA* 1995;274:562–569.
14. Hu WT, Wijdicks EF. Sudden coma due to acute bilateral M1 occlusion. *Mayo Clin Proc* 2007;82:1155.
15. Kim J, Kemp S, Kullas K, et al. Injury patterns in patients who "talk and die." *J Clin Neurosci* 2013;20:1697–1701.
16. Kolias AG, Kirkpatrick PJ, Hutchinson PJ. Decompressive craniotomy: past, present, and future. *Nat Rev Neurol*. 2013;9:405–415.
17. Krantz T, Thisted B, Strøm J, Sørensen MB. Acute carbon monoxide poisoning. *Acta Anaesthesiol Scand* 1988;32:278–282.
18. Leão M. Valproate as a cause of hyperammonemia in heterozygotes with ornithine-transcarbamylase deficiency. *Neurology* 1995;45:593–594.
19. Maramattom BV, Bahn MM, Wijdicks EFM. Which patient fares worse after early deterioration due to swelling from hemispheric stroke? *Neurology* 2004;63:2142–2145.
20. Mégarbane B, Borron SW, Baud FJ. Current recommendations for treatment of severe toxic alcohol poisonings. *Intensive Care Med* 2005;31:189–195.
21. Nice A, Leikin JB, Maturen A, et al. Toxidrome recognition to improve efficiency of emergency urine drug screens. *Ann Emerg Med* 1988;17:676–680.
22. Rabinstein AA, Atkinson JL, Wijdicks EFM. Emergency craniotomy in patients worsening due to expanded cerebral hematoma: to what purpose? *Neurology* 2002;58:1367–1372.
23. Reed CE, Driggs MF, Foote CC. Acute barbiturate intoxication: a study of 300 cases based on a physiologic system of classification of the severity of the intoxication. *Ann Intern Med* 1952;37:290–303.
24. St Louis EK, Wijdicks EFM, Li H. Predicting neurologic deterioration in patients with cerebellar hematomas. *Neurology* 1998;51:1364–1369.

25. Stefini R, Latronico N, Cornali C, Rasulo F, Bollati A. Emergent decompressive craniec-tomy in patients with fixed dilated pupils due to cerebral venous and dural sinus thrombo-sis: report of three cases. *Neurosurgery* 1999;45:626–629.

26. Wijdicks EFM, Bamlet WR, Maramattom BV, Manno EM, McClelland RL. Validation of a new coma scale: The FOUR score. *Ann Neurol* 2005;58:585–593.

27. Wijdicks EFM. The Comatose Patient, second edition. New York, Oxford University Press, 2014.

28. Wijdicks EFM. The bare essentials: coma. *Pract Neurol* 2010;10:51–60.

2

When Seizures Continue

Any seizure is a reason for concern. Most patients with a second seizure will be treated with an intravenous loading dose of (fos)phenytoin or levetiracetam after a single dose of lorazepam does not stop the seizures. It is usually when the third seizure occurs that the entire clinical picture changes. A seizure usually lasts several minutes, and any seizure that is longer than this arbitrary time period should prompt aggressive seizure termination and close monitoring of the patient. There is a general agreement among epileptologists that a long duration of a single seizure may indicate higher proclivity for another seizure and even status epilepticus. There is also a sense that a refractory condition can rapidly emerge—more rapid than previously thought.[56]

Seizures typically stop, but it is largely unknown what biochemical mechanism is at work that stops a seizure. Terminating mechanisms have been proposed— and will be mentioned here—but in clinical practice it is mainly predicated on the time needed for an antiepileptic drug to reach peak plasma concentration. Although the true mechanisms of status epilepticus after a single seizure are unknown, there are profound changes in neuronal physiology and architectural structure, mostly in the limbic system. The anatomical changes are rapid, leaving little time to spare. This would indicate that initial polytherapy rather than one single drug approach may be needed to avoid refractory seizures.

How do we recognize established status epilepticus? What are the drugs of choice? Is it all just randomly trying after the first antiepileptic drugs fail, or can we make any sense out of all those algorithms? Is one drug enough or do we need a one-two punch? This chapter discusses how to manage recurrent seizures and the evolution to status epilepticus, including transition to refractory status epilepticus. Status epilepticus may be difficult to treat if significant comorbidities are present, in which case prior outcome may be more likely.

Principles

One might think that epileptogenesis and self-termination may be simple on and off switches.[29] Such is not the case. To understand recurrent seizures and status epilepticus, several fundamentals—without going into too much detail—have to be understood.

The first core principle relates to our current understanding of ongoing seizure activity. Anatomically, one of the proven pathways is so-called receptor trafficking, which pertains to changes in the function of gamma-aminobutyric acid (GABA) and N-methyl-D-aspartate (NMDA) receptors.[35-37] With ongoing seizures, the GABA receptors reduce in numbers and are internalized into endocytic vessels and destroyed, which results in decreased GABAergic inhibition.[14] On the other hand, there is increased transport of the NMDA receptors to the synaptic membrane, resulting in an increased number of excitatory NMDA receptors per synapse. Therefore, lack of inhibition and increased excitation as a result of interplay of these two receptors may perpetuate sustained seizures or status epilepticus (Figure 2.1).[5,34,43] This observation is important to keep in mind, because therapy can be more rational if it approaches different targets at the same time. One could see that a combination of a benzodiazepine with an NMDA antagonist (e.g., ketamine) may improve control of seizures.

Physiologically, status epilepticus presents as neurons that are prolongedly depolarized with sustained potassium efflux. Eventually energy shutdown occurs as a result of increased ATP utilization to restore ionic gradients across the

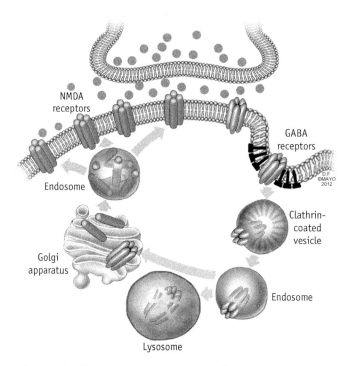

Figure 2.1 Changes in GABA and NMDA receptors after continuing seizures.
(Adapted from Wasterlain CG, Treiman DM. *Status Epilepticus: Mechanisms and Management.* Cambridge (MA), MIT Press, 2006.)

membranes. There is also an increased synchrony across neurons, which can be seen on EEG that shows progressive increase in amplitude and slowing of the discharge. It has been hypothesized that this synchrony activates sodium calcium inflow and eventually will silence neuronal firing.[53]

The second core principle is to understand the mechanisms of status epilepticus becoming refractory to drug treatment—this is far more complicated. One prevailing theory is that loss of GABAergic receptor density also decreases the effectiveness of GABAergic drugs such as benzodiazepines or barbiturates in controlling seizures. In addition, the extracellular ionic environment may play a role, and there has even been a suggestion that normally inhibitory GABA currents may become excitatory if there is significant change in chlorine concentrations.[30] Refractory status epilepticus can also be caused by an inflammatory process, with opening of the blood-brain barrier resulting in leakage of higher potassium levels during excitation. Mitochondrial collapse has been proposed and may result in opening apoptosis pathways. Such a concept potentially justifies treatment with high dose corticosteroids.

Essentially, there is an excitation/inhibition imbalance. There is a down-regulation of GABA receptors, which may explain the decrease in efficacy of benzodiazepines within the first 30 minutes of seizure onset. The excitatory activity results in an increase in NMDA; because these receptors are activated, the glutamate increases, which in turn increases intracellular calcium, resulting in injury and possibly promoting seizures. The increased calcium results in caspase activation and apoptotic pathways. This is the rationale for NMDA receptor antagonists and also the rationale for using one in a late stage of status epilepticus. Therefore, one approach to status epilepticus is to simultaneously target several receptors, not only GABA or NMDA—this would theoretically lead to using drugs in a lower, less harmful dose.[65,66]

A third core principle is that seizures damage the brain, and the key is to be found via neuroimaging, autopsy data, and reproducible animal experiments. Structures such as the insular, piriform, entorhinal, and prelimbic cortices are showing neuronal cell loss or drop out with parahippocampal gyrus inclusively involved, although it is not the very first structure that loses neurons.[32]

The EEG changes and becomes disorganized. EEG stages of status epilepticus have been suggested (Table 2.1).[59] These EEG stages might be useful, but eventually they may culminate in generalized periodic epileptiform discharges (GPEDs). The EEG will show little variability in frequency, amplitude, and morphology, and making a distinction between ictal and interictal activity may become very difficult. Periodic epileptiform discharges in EEGs of patients who are in status epilepticus are considered indicative of poor outcome, but it can also represent the underlying etiology.

A fourth principle is that seizures damage other organs. Status epilepticus, it turns out, results in a dramatic physiologic response, some of which is damaging. A major temperature increase, reaching hyperthermic levels (40°C), may occur.

Table 2.1 **EEG Stages of Status Epilepticus**

Stage 1	Discrete seizures
Stage 2	Merging seizures with waxing and waning amplitudes and frequencies
Stage 3	Continuous ictal activity
Stage 4	Continuous ictal activity interrupted by flat periods
Stage 5	Generalized periodic complexes on a flat background

Source: From reference 62.

Well set-up animal experiments clearly demonstrated that untreated hyperthermia may cause more areas of neuronal necrosis; and, again, increased excitatory neurotransmitter release was observed during hyperthermic periods. This combination of fever and seizures is underappreciated by clinicians, who should find ways early on to cool patients who actively seize.[24] Another relevant change is the massive increase in catecholamines, leading to hyperglycemia and cardiac arrhythmias that may be life threatening or cause hypotension. Heart muscle is not spared, and an apical ballooning syndrome has been well documented—very similar to a "broken heart" stress cardiomyopathy. Furthermore, lactic acidosis produced by anaerobic metabolism in jerking overworked muscles may play some role in cardiac arrhythmias.

In Practice

Status epilepticus is a brain in synchronized chaos. Perhaps the same can be said of treatment algorithms with drugs going in and out of favor and constant changes in treatment approach with little new drug breakthroughs.[57] Regardless, physicians have an obligation to press on quickly with treatment but there should be some sense of proportionality. The first-line agent of status epilepticus is established, and suggestions have been proposed for when the first-line approach is not successful.[5,10,18,22,38,51,52] (Management of status epilepticus in children is difficult for several reasons, well covered in several reviews and not considered here.[10,11,49,59,69])

The Neurocritical Care Society has recently published an approach based on a consensus statement.[4] The major recommendations reflect current practices and include: (1) rapid treatment of clinical and electrographic seizures; (2) IV lorazepam, intramuscular midazolam, or rectal diazepam as first-line drugs; (3) IV (fos)phenytoin, valproic acid, or levetiracetam as second-line drugs; (4) anesthetic drugs should be titrated to burst suppression or isoelectric EEG; (5) duration of treatment should be at least 24 hours before weaning from anesthetic drugs; (6) maintenance drugs should be provided before weaning; and (7) transfer to a neurosciences intensive care unit with experience in long-term management.

The first line of treatment in status epilepticus or rapidly recurrent seizures may undergo changes. For many practitioners, it remains an almost unwatchable experience when seizures continue during the "long" infusion of fosphenytoin and often wonder in frustration if there is nothing better, or whether rapid intubation with an anesthetic is not a more reasonable option. Also of interest is the recent appearance of intramuscular or buccal midazolam as a treatment for status epilepticus, already widely used outside the hospital. There also has been a move toward rapidly escalating treatment with intravenous valproic acid in a dose of 30 mg/kg. In fact, valproic acid may terminate seizures in two-thirds of the patients as compared to phenytoin's success rate of under 50%.[13] A combination of valproic acid and phenytoin could possibly be effective in nearly 90% of the patients.[13]

For now, treatment starts with repeated doses of 4 mg of lorazepam. When seizures are not controlled with a first and second dose, lorazepam is soon followed by phenytoin or (fos)phenytoin (intravenous loading 20–25 mg/kg.)[4,16] In Europe, intravenous clonazepam 0.015 mg/kg is combined with phenytoin. Other less accepted proposals use a combination of IV diazepam with ketamine and valproate. The IV dose of diazepam would be 1 mg/kg with ketamine 10 mg/kg and valproic acid 30 mg/kg.

The treatment of seizures probably should start before reaching the hospital, and significant improvement has been made in the ultra-early care of status epilepticus. Intramuscular midazolam, administered by paramedics in patients who had seizures lasting more than 5 minutes, was found to terminate seizures in 73% as opposed to 63% in the intravenous lorazepam treatment group.[58] As an alternative, nasal or buccal midazolam may be used and these are absorbed more quickly than intramuscular midazolam.[2] It is not uncommon to see intranasal or buccal administration blown or spat out by a seizing patient. Thus, the development of intramuscular auto-injectors for midazolam will improve the prehospital management of status epilepticus.

Ketamine is a drug of interest and may provide a new treatment option not only late in status epilepticus but also early on. Ketamine does not have any cardiac depressive properties and does not cause major hypotension. Even in patients who are not intubated, a single dose of ketamine does not necessarily result in emergency intubation.[24,54]

Treatment of status epilepticus often requires endotracheal intubation with mechanical ventilation and initiation of intravenous anesthetic agents titrated to control seizures. This is often a key moment where a new phase of treatment starts.[67] Monitoring using continuous EEG provides essential information and allows deep sedation, resulting in varying degrees of burst suppression. The control of seizures is dependent on the degree of EEG suppression. EEG monitoring therefore can show that the EEG is sufficiently suppressed and that no

further seizures occur intermittently. In patients for whom endotracheal intubation is problematic, there are several antiepileptic drugs that can be considered
that do not result in depression of the breathing drive or upper airway collapse
from sedation. These include intravenous lacosamide, intravenous valproic acid,
and subanesthetic doses of intravenous phenobarbital.

Most protocols do progress through stages. One approach is shown in Fig. 2.2.
There is insufficient evidence to recommend one anesthetic agent over another.
Options include valproic acid, midazolam, propofol, or a barbiturate (pentobarbital or phenobarbital).[7,13] Patients may develop tachyphylaxis to midazolam, neces-
sitating higher doses or a change of therapy.

Propofol modulates GABA receptors and has an effect similar to barbiturates
or midazolam.[48] The drug has significant potential for toxicity, including the risk
of propofol infusion syndrome, which results in metabolic acidosis, rhabdomyolysis, bradycardia, and cardiovascular collapse. Albeit very uncommon, many
patients die from propofol infusion syndrome, which is usually only found in
patients with a higher dose (often more than 200 mg/kg/min) and long infusion
times (defined as 3 days or more). Propofol infusion syndrome was also found to
be more common in patients on a ketogenic diet but only if there is an associated acidosis.[25] Therefore, while use of propofol for refractory status epilepticus
is widespread, we have become cautious about using the drug after two cases of
propofol infusion syndrome resulted in deaths. (Surprisingly, many reviews on
status epilepticus allow a high dose of propofol [up to 10 mg/kg/h].)[51,55]

When electrographic status has been controlled for 48 hours and therapeutic
levels of at least two conventional antiepileptic drugs have been achieved, an
attempt is made to wean from the anesthetic agent. If clinical or electrographic
status epilepticus recurs on weaning from the anesthetic agent, the drug should

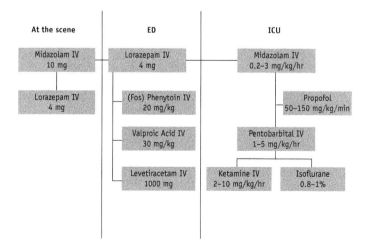

Figure 2.2 Guide to treatment of status epilepticus.

simply be resumed, and additional therapeutic options may be considered. This cycle of weaning and then reinstituting anesthesia if seizures recur may occur frequently. Other drugs may be used when repeated attempts to liberate the patient from a barbiturate infusion result in recurrent status epilepticus. Unfortunately, some of these drugs result in excellent control of seizures but only transiently with recurrence of the epileptic pattern on weaning. There is efficacy reported with topiramate[61] and with the use of intravenous lacosamide[17]. Bolus doses of lacosamide—2 mg/kg after three or more standard antiepileptic drugs have been ineffective—have been proposed.[17,21] Levetiracetam is another emerging drug for status epilepticus that can be administered intravenously and may be an important adjunctive therapy.[3] At least one study suggested that with a median dose of 3,500 mg IV levetiracetam could result in a success rate of 72%.

The use of corticosteroids or immunotherapy provides significant options in patients with autoimmune encephalitis (Chapter 5), but it also may have a place in refractory status epilepticus.[34] The dose is unclear, and in autoimmune encephalitis corticosteroids are often combined with IV immunoglobulins.

A final option is to proceed with cortical resection of the epileptic focus, which first needs to be identified with single photon emission computed tomography. This is usually only considered after weeks and even months of failed medical management.[31,44] Another option is vagal nerve stimulation, but there is only anecdotal experience.[45,63,69]

Knowing these options (Table 2.2), what can be done? Once status epilepticus becomes refractory, propofol and midazolam can be considered. Propofol acts on GABA receptors but may also inhibit NMDA receptors.[28] However, midazolam is purely targeted to the benzodiazepine site of the GABA receptors. Midazolam is far less effective than propofol.[6,7] However, each of these agents should be tried. The next step would be to consider ketamine. Ketamine is used in a loading dose of 1 mg/kg followed by an infusion of 2–10 mg/kg/hr, again titrating to burst-suppression pattern.[28,42] Ketamine might be synergistic with benzodiazepines, but using the combination may lead to hypotension and may be rate limiting.

The decision to proceed with inhalational anesthetics using isoflurane requires a detailed preparation and a daily anesthesiologist visit to monitor its administration. Although a large anesthesia machine will take up much space, and a good outlet for exhaled gases should be found, it is remarkably simple to set up, and a minimum alveolar concentration of 0.2–1% is often enough to fully suppress the EEG. Anesthesia over multiple days may be concerning, and we found that the MRI scans can become transiently abnormal if a high or prolonged dose of isoflurane is used.[12]

One last option is to lower the core body temperature. There is a significant interest in early treatment of status epilepticus with hypothermia. Several studies of aggressive hypothermia using superficial or endovascular cooling to 32°C–35°C

Table 2.2 **Antiepileptic Drugs in Status Epilepticus**

Drug	Dose	Infusion Rate	Precautions and Interactions
Lorazepam	4 mg IV	1–2 min	Sedation Slow to clear in hepatic failure
Phenytoin or Fosphenytoin	20 mg/kg IV load, mixed in normal saline 20 mg/kg IV	50 mg/min 100–150 mg/min	Bradycardia, hypotension, Slow to clear in hepatic failure Drug interactions Hypotension in elderly
Valproic acid	30 mg/kg IV	30 min–1 h	Caution with impaired hepatic function Hyperammonemic syndrome (rare)
Levetiracetam	1000 mg IV	Undefined	Minimal No major drug interactions
Propofol	1 mg/kg IV	50–200 mcg/kg/min, titrate to burst-suppression on EEG	Hypotension Propofol infusion syndrome (rare)
Midazolam	0.2 mg/kg IV	0.2–3 mg/kg/h	Hypotension, Tachyphylaxis
Phenobarbital	15–20 mg/kg IV	100 mg/min	Hypotension Respiratory depression
Pentobarbital	5 mg/kg IV	1–5 mg/kg/h	Hypotension Metabolic acidosis (osmolar gap)
Ketamine	1 mg/kg IV	2–10 mg/kg/h	Hypotension
Topiramate	300–1,600 mg	Only oral	Metabolic acidosis
Lacosamide	200–400 mg IV	60 mg/min	Rash, Pruritis

Source: Adapted from reference 19.

did find more effective control seizures.[8,15,46] Hypothermia is easy to use, and often does not require additional treatment for shivering due to the already high dose of antiepileptic drugs.

A ketogenic diet can be considered using a special formula (usually 4:1 lipid-to-nonlipid ratio), but because many day-to-day drugs have carbohydrates, it is challenging to maintain ketoacidosis.[41] Moreover, a ketogenic diet may take several days to become effective. The diet is also associated with liver function abnormalities, pancreatitis, hyperlipidemia, and gastroesophageal reflux (due to prolonged gastric emptying time with high-fat diets that may lead to aspiration) if used for longer periods.

In each of these situations, continuous EEG is used to guide the depth of anesthesia aiming at absent seizure activity, accepting a few sharp waves and generalized periodic epileptiform discharges and often down to burst suppression or isoelectric EEG patterns. A most contentious issue is when to stop treatment of status epilepticus after patients have been treated unsuccessfully for many months[60] (see also volume *Communicating Prognosis*). Diffusion-weighted MRI scans may show significant atrophy over time, and this finding might indicate a poor prognosis. The atrophy should be more generalized than purely hippocampal, involving the mesial temporal structure, because these abnormalities are potentially reversible.

The cause of death is sometimes a major medical complication leading to cardiac arrest; but much more often, the mere fact that all efforts were in vain for many months may lead the family to decide to withdraw intensive care support. It appears that once third-line (anesthetic) drugs and vasopressors are needed, the prognosis changes.[26] Many patients die or stay severely disabled. Mortality, therefore, in status epilepticus (as in many other neurocatastrophes) is a result of coming to grips with the futility of management. Clinical experience suggests that patients with refractory status should be treated aggressively early on, with treatment of the underlying etiology (when known), "ample" treatment time should be allowed, and therapeutic options should be exhausted before futility is determined. What constitutes "ample" treatment time is a clinical judgment and is different for each patient. It may be based on premorbid factors such as functional status and whether the underlying etiology is expected to be progressive or untreatable.[1]

By the Way

- Status epilepticus requires an aggressive, rapid approach using appropriate doses of drugs and quickly changing to another drug if there is no effect
- Status epilepticus has a better outcome in patients with known seizures
- Status epilepticus may become untreatable early on
- Status epilepticus may resolve after several months of treatment
- Status epilepticus initially requires sufficient treatment to achieve an EEG with burst-suppression or isoelectric pattern

Status Epilepticus by the Numbers

- ~80% of status epilepticus treated with anesthetic drugs need vasopressors
- ~75% of status epilepticus is controlled with lorazepam and phenytoin
- ~50% of status epilepticus is controlled with lorazepam
- ~30% of status epilepticus occurs in chronic epilepsy
- ~15% of status epilepticus is never controlled

Putting It All Together

- Achieve rapid control of seizures even if intubation, anesthetic drugs, and vasopressors are needed
- Polytherapy may result in better control
- There is no convincing preference for the available second-line drugs
- Continuous EEG monitoring is necessary to guide therapy and to prove no interval seizure activity
- Hypothermia and ketogenic diet are unproven last resorts

References

1. Alvarez V, Januel JM, Burnand B, Rossetti AO. Role of comorbidities in outcome prediction after status epilepticus. *Epilepsia* 2012;53:e89–e92.
2. Anderson GD, Saneto RP. Current oral and non-oral routes of antiepileptic drug delivery. *Adv Drug Deliv Rev* 2012;64:911–918.
3. Berning S, Boesebeck F, van Baalen A, Kellinghaus C. Intravenous levetiracetam as treatment for status epilepticus. *J Neurol* 2009;256:1634–1642.
4. Brophy GM, Bell R, Claassen J, et al. Guidelines for the evaluation and management of status epilepticus. *NeurocritCare* 2012;17:3–23.
5. Chen JW, Wasterlain CG. Status epilepticus: pathophysiology and management in adults. *Lancet Neurol* 2006;5:246–256.
6. Claassen J, Hirsch LJ, Emerson RG, et al. Continuous EEG monitoring and midazolam infusion for refractory nonconvulsive status epilepticus. *Neurology* 2001;57:1036–1042.
7. Claassen J, Hirsch LJ, Emerson RG, Mayer SA. Treatment of refractory status epilepticus with pentobarbital, propofol, or midazolam: a systematic review. *Epilepsia* 2002;43:146–153.
8. Corry JJ, Dhar R, Murphy T, Diringer MN. Hypothermia for refractory status epilepticus. *Neurocrit Care* 2008;9:189–197.
9. Delanty N, French JA, Labar DR, Pedley TA, Rowan AJ. Status epilepticus arising de novo in hospitalized patients: an analysis of 41 patients. *Seizure* 2001;10:116–119.
10. Fernandez A, Claassen J. Refractory status epilepticus. *Curr Opin Crit Care* 2012;18:127–131.
11. Friedman J. Emergency management of the pediatric patient with generalized convulsive status epilepticus. *Paediatr Child Health* 2011;16:91–104.
12. Fugate JE, Burns JD, Wijdicks EFM, et al. Prolonged high-dose isoflurane for refractory status epilepticus: is it safe? *Anesth Analg* 2010;111:1520–1524.

13. Gilad R, Izkovitz N, Dabby R, et al. Treatment of status epilepticus and acute repetitive seizures with i.v. valproic acid vs phenytoin. *Acta Neurol Scand* 2008;118:296–300.
14. Goodkin HP, Yeh JL, Kapur J. Status epilepticus increases the intracellular accumulation of GABAA receptors. *J Neurosci* 2005;25:5511–5520.
15. Guilliams K, Rosen M, Buttram S, et al. Hypothermia for pediatric refractory status epilepticus. *Epilepsia*. 2013;54:1586–1594.
16. Hirsch LJ. Intramuscular versus intravenous benzodiazepines for prehospital treatment of status epilepticus. *N Engl J Med* 2012;366:659–660.
17. Höfler J, Trinka E. Lacosamide as a new treatment option in status epilepticus. *Epilepsia* 2013;54(3):393–404.
18. Holtkamp M, Tong X, Walker MC. Propofol in subanesthetic doses terminates status epilepticus in a rodent model. *Ann Neurol* 2001;49:260–263.
19. Hunter G, Young GB. Status epilepticus: a review, with emphasis on refractory cases. *Can J Neurol Sci* 2012;39:157–169.
20. Iyer VN, Hoel R, Rabinstein AA. Propofol infusion syndrome in patients with refractory status epilepticus: an 11-year clinical experience. *Crit Care Med* 2009;37:3024–3030.
21. Jain V, Harvey AS. Treatment of refractory tonic status epilepticus with intravenous lacosamide. *Epilepsia* 2012;53:761–762.
22. Kälviäinen R. Status epilepticus treatment guidelines. *Epilepsia* 2007;48:99–102.
23. Kapur J, Lothman EW. NMDA receptor activation mediates the loss of GABAergic inhibition induced by recurrent seizures. *Epilepsy Res* 1990;5:103–111.
24. Kofke WA, Bloom MJ, Van Cott A, Brenner RP. Electrographic tachyphylaxis to etomidate and ketamine used for refractory status epilepticus controlled with isoflurane. *J Neurosurg Anesthesiol* 1997;9:269–272.
25. Kossoff E. The fat is in the fire: ketogenic diet for refractory status epilepticus. *Epilepsy Curr* 2011;11:88–89.
26. Kowalski RG, Ziai WC, Rees RN, et al. Third-line antiepileptic therapy and outcome in status epilepticus: The impact of vasopressor use and prolonged mechanical ventilation. *Crit Care Med* 2012;40:2677–2684.
27. Kowski AB, Kanaan H, Schmitt FC, Holtkamp M. Deep hypothermia terminates status epilepticus—an experimental study. *Brain Res* 2012;1446:119–126.
28. Kramer AH. Early ketamine to treat refractory status epilepticus. *Neurocrit Care* 2012;16:299–305.
29. Lado F, Moshe SL. How do seizures stop? *Epilepsia* 2008;49:1651–1664.
30. Lamsa K, Taira T. Use-dependent shift from inhibitory to excitatory GABAA receptor action in SP-O interneurons in the rat hippocampal CA3 area. *J Neurophysiol* 2003;90:1983–1995.
31. Lhatoo SD, Alexopoulos AV. The surgical treatment of status epilepticus. *Epilepsia* 2007;48:61–65.
32. Macdonald RL, Kapur J. Acute cellular alterations in the hippocampus after status epilepticus. *Epilepsia* 1999;40:S9–S20.
33. Maeda T, Hashizume K, Tanaka T. Effect of hypothermia on kainic acid-induced limbic seizures: an electroencephalographic and 14C-deoxyglucose autoradiographic study. *Brain Res* 1999;818:228–235.
34. Marchi N, Granata T, Freri E, et al. Efficacy of anti-inflammatory therapy in a model of acute seizures and in a population of pediatric drug resistant epileptics. *PLoS One* 2011;28:e18200.
35. Mazarati AM, Baldwin RA, Sankar R, Wasterlain CG. Time-dependent decrease in the effectiveness of antiepileptic drugs during the course of self-sustaining status epilepticus. *Brain Res* 1998;814:179–185.
36. Mazarati AM, Wasterlain CG. N-methyl-D-asparate receptor antagonists abolish the maintenance phase of self-sustaining status epilepticus in rat. *Neurosci Lett* 1999;265:187–190.
37. Mazarati AM, Wasterlain CG. N-methyl-D-asparate receptor antagonists abolish the maintenance phase of self-sustaining status epilepticus in rat. *Neurosci Lett* 1999;265:187–190.

38. Meierkord H, Boon P, Engelsen B, et al. EFNS guideline on the management of status epilepticus in adults. *Eur J Neurol* 2010;17:348–355.
39. Mirsattari SM, Sharpe MD, Young GB. Treatment of refractory status epilepticus with inhalational anesthetic agents isoflurane and desflurane. *Arch Neurol* 2004;61:1254–1259.
40. Misra UK, Kalita J, Patel R. Sodium valproate vs phenytoin in status epilepticus: a pilot study. *Neurology* 2006;67:340–342.
41. Nam SH, Lee BL, Lee CG, et al. The role of ketogenic diet in the treatment of refractory status epilepticus. *Epilepsia* 2011;52:e181–e184.
42. Nathan B, Smith TL, Bleck TB. The use of ketamine in the treatment of refractory status epilepticus. *Neurology* 2002;3:A197.
43. Naylor DE, Liu H, Wasterlain CG. Trafficking of GABA (A) receptors, loss of inhibition, and a mechanism for pharmacoresistance in status epilepticus. *J Neurosci* 2005;25:7724–7733.
44. Ng YT, Bristol RE, Schrader DV, Smith KA. The role of neurosurgery in status epilepticus. *Neurocrit Care* 2007;7:86–91.
45. O'Neill BR, Valeriano J, Synowiec A, et al. Refractory status epilepticus treated with vagal nerve stimulation: case report. *Neurosurgery* 2011;69:E1172–E1175.
46. Orlowski JP, Erenberg G, Lueders H, Cruse RP. Hypothermia and barbiturate coma for refractory status epilepticus. *Crit Care Med* 1984;12:367–372.
47. Patil B, Oware A. De-novo simple partial status epilepticus presenting as Wernicke's aphasia. *Seizure* 2012;21:219–222.
48. Power KN, Flaatten H, Gilhus NE, Engelsen BA. Propofol treatment in adult refractory status epilepticus. Mortality risk and outcome. *Epilepsy Res* 2011;94:53–60.
49. Riviello JJ Jr, Ashwal S, Hirtz D, et al. Practice parameter: diagnostic assessment of the child with status epilepticus (an evidence-based review): report of the Quality Standards Subcommittee of the American Academy of Neurology and the Practice Committee of the Child Neurology Society. *Neurology* 2006;67:1542–1550.
50. Robakis TK, Hirsch LJ. Literature review, case report, and expert discussion of prolonged refractory status epilepticus. *Neurocrit Care* 2006;4:35–46.
51. Rossetti AO, Lowenstein DH. Management of refractory status epilepticus in adults: still more questions than answers. *Lancet Neurol* 2011;10:922–930.
52. Rossetti AO, Milligan TA, Vulliémoz S, et al. A randomized trial for the treatment of refractory status epilepticus. *Neurocrit Care* 2011;14:4–10.
53. Schindler K, Elger CE, Lehnertz K. Increasing synchronization may promote seizure termination: evidence from status epilepticus. *Clin Neurophysiol* 2007;118:1955–1968.
54. Sheth RD, Gidal IS. Refractory status epilepticus: response to ketamine. *Neurology* 1998;51:1765–1766.
55. Shorvon S, Ferlisi M. The outcome of therapies in refractory and super-refractory convulsive status epilepticus and recommendations for therapy. *Brain* 2012;135:2314–2328.
56. Shorvon S, Ferlisi M. The treatment of super-refractory status epilepticus: a critical review of available therapies and a clinical treatment protocol. *Brain* 2011;134:2802–2818.
57. Shorvon S. The historical evolution of, and the paradigms shifts in, the therapy of convulsive status epilepticus over the past 150 years. *Epilepsia*. 2013;54 Suppl 6:64–67.
58. Silbergleit R, Durkalski V, Lowenstein D, et al. Intramuscular versus intravenous therapy for prehospital status epilepticus. *N Engl J Med* 2012;366:591–600.
59. Sofou K, Kristjánsdóttir R, Papachatzakis NE, Ahmadzadeh A, Uvebrant P. Management of prolonged seizures and status epilepticus in childhood: a systematic review. *J Child Neurol* 2009;24:918–926.
60. Standley K, Abdulmassih R, Benbadis S. Good outcome is possible after months of refractory convulsive status epilepticus: lesson learned. *Epilepsia* 2012;53:e17–e20.
61. Synowiec AS, Yandora KA, Yenugadhati V, et al. The efficacy of topiramate in adult refractory status epilepticus: experience of a tertiary care center. *Epilepsy Res* 2012;98:232–237.
62. Treiman DM, Walton NY, Kendrick C. A progressive sequence of electroencephalographic changes during generalized convulsive status epilepticus. *Epilepsy Res* 1990;5:49–60.

63. Valentín A, Nguyen HQ, Skupenova AM, et al. Centromedian thalamic nuclei deep brain stimulation in refractory status epilepticus. *Brain Stimul* 2012;5:594–598.

64. Verellen RM, Cavazos JE. Pathophysiological considerations of seizures, epilepsy, and status epilepticus in the elderly. *Aging Dis* 2011;2:278–285.

65. Voss LJ, Sleigh JW, Barnard JPM, Kirsch HE. The howling cortex: seizures and general anesthetic drugs. *Anesth Analg* 2008;107:1689–1703.

66. Wasterlain CG, Baldwin R, Naylor DE, et al. Rational polytherapy in the treatment of acute seizures and status epilepticus. *Epilepsia* 2011;52 Suppl 8:70–71.

67. Wijdicks EFM. The multifaceted care of status epilepticus. *Epilepsia* 2013;54 Suppl 6:61–63.

68. Winston KRM, Levisohn P, Miller BR, Freeman J. Vagal nerve stimulation for status epilepticus. *Pediatr Neurosurg* 2001;34:190–192.

69. Yoong M, Chin RF, Scott RC. Management of convulsive status epilepticus in children. *Arch Dis Child Educ Pract Ed* 2009;94:1–9.

3

Judging Severity of
Traumatic Brain Injury

Forceful impact to the head may cause movement of the brain within the skull. Rather than protecting the brain, the skull causes injury that may result in localized or diffuse brain lesions. An initial clinical assessment first divides traumatic brain injury (TBI) into penetrating versus nonpenetrating injury, with penetrating head injury mostly a result of gunshot wounds. Obviously penetrating brain injury is far more injurious, as is exposure to an explosive detonation. Depending on the nature of the injury, trauma to the brain may not be the only lesion and there may be other bodily harm that is not immediately clinically apparent.

There are urgent priorities in the assessment of a patient with a TBI besides judging the type of injury. The presence of multisystem injury such as injury to the spine, chest, abdomen, or pelvis needs to be considered, followed by immediate stabilization of the patient before surgical or neurosurgical decisions are made.

The most deceptive situation is the wide awake patient with no apparent injury and minimal findings on CT scan. Some of these tiny hemorrhages may later blossom to more profound contusions and the patient may deteriorate hours later.[23,44] Prior use of warfarin or antiplatelet agents may play an important role in later worsening.

Over a million patients are seen in emergency departments in the United States each year and several hundred thousand are admitted for management.[14,46] How do we recognize "high-risk" patients? What constitutes a comprehensive neurologic assessment, and what are the immediate pitfalls? What are the fundamental principles of intervention in traumatic head injury that should be known to any physician working in these locations? What are adequate resources to appropriately resuscitate these patients? This chapter discusses these difficult judgments.

Principles

The brain and the vascular structures within it cannot resist much injury. There are many ways to classify TBI if we want to improve triage or need to consider specific

Table 3.1 **Types of Traumatic Brain Injury***

- Diffuse axonal injury
- Hemorrhagic contusions
- Blast injury
- Penetrating injury
- Brainstem injury
- Acute subdural hematoma
- Acute epidural hematoma

*Combinations are common

intervention. TBI can be categorized by mechanism (closed or penetrating), by injury (parenchymal, extraparenchymal, skull fractures), and by severity (coma or transient loss of consciousness)[16,29,33] (Table 3.1). Injury can also be due to secondary insults from systemic complications or due to injury to arteries causing stroke.

The mechanism of trauma can also be further categorized as contact forces or acceleration–deceleration forces. Each of these transmitting forces has been replicated in animal models set up to study its impact. The biomechanics of tissue injury are, at its simplest, tension causing compression or stretch, or shear due to misshaping of the soft brain and vascular tissues. In general, it has been recognized that force alone cannot explain the severity of injury, and concussion effect is largely related to rotational changes that produce shearing strains. The physics associated with a blast injury to the brain are far more complex and involve the direct effect of a shock wave, but also possible penetrating injury from flying debris or impact associated with victims flying through the air.[12,19] The main biomechanical mechanisms are shown in Figure 3.1.

A direct hit to the skull can result in injury at the site, but also at other sites due to some movement of the brain against the bony protuberances of the anterior middle fossa or against the hard falx. Acceleration or deceleration results in

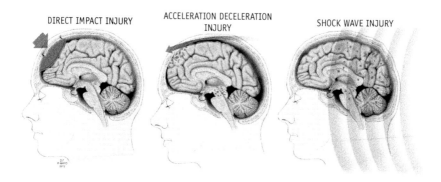

Figure 3.1 Forces that cause traumatic brain injury.

tissue shearing, mostly in areas where there is highest angular force. Typically these areas are at the junction between the gray and white matter, but also in the rostral brainstem and this explains the location of these lesions in more severe injuries. Injuries also impact on axonal projections in the corpus callosum and in the gray and white matter junction of the central and anterior frontal and temporal lobes.[5] Injury may be more simply due to compression and shift (epidural or subdural hematoma). Blast injury causes multiple minute tearing of axons and blood vessels. These lesions are widespread and the extent of the damage is often difficult to calibrate.

The neuropathology of TBI is diverse and can also be divided into primary (the abnormality at the time of impact) or secondary injury (the abnormalities evolving later, including brain swelling and its consequences). In primary axonal injury, so-called breaking of axonal microtubules is observed.[34] At multiple sites there is twisting and misalignment of these microtubules and they interrupt axonal transport, eventually also inducing swelling and degeneration. Axons of the white matter are particularly vulnerable to injury, specifically the unmyelinated fibers. These axons eventually undergo Wallerian degeneration. Tearing is histologically recognized by the appearance of numerous retraction balls at the ends of interrupted nerve fibers.[35,47,55]

TBI also changes the normally balanced cerebral metabolism and circulation. The changes are not entirely understood, but there are a few common themes. Cerebral metabolism in comatose patients is half of what it should be, and cerebrovascular reactivity may be impaired—usually preserving the CO_2 reactivity. All of these changes are influenced by changes in intracranial pressure (further details can be found in another volume of the series, *Recognizing Brain Injury*).

It has been well established that other, more delayed, responses can occur beyond the initial changes on a cellular level.[10,11,58] These secondary insults are just as important as the impact and may even be worse. Factors such as poor oxygenation (i.e., inability to secure an airway and administer oxygen) and inadequate fluid resuscitation (i.e., significant blood loss) contribute to a more significant injury.

Furthermore, post-TBI cerebral vasospasm has been recognized as a cause of deterioration and may even emerge in patients with relatively small brain contusions.[51] There appears to be a relation between admission core body temperature and development of post-traumatic vasospasm resulting in speculation that it is a manifestation of systemic inflammatory response syndrome. The presence of traumatic subarachnoid hemorrhage does not appear to be correlated to traumatic vasospasm.

Another cause of worsening in initially seemingly stable patients is the development of contusions, often bifrontal contusions, and there is usually extensive edema.[40,44,57] These blossoming contusions may occur up to a week after the initial impact in most patients, but there is a marked variation in clinical presentation.[9,40] Some patients rapidly worsen ("talk, deteriorate and die"); others

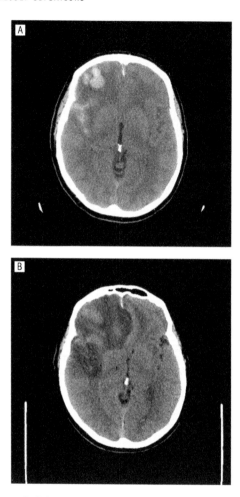

Figure 3.2 CT scans with delayed temporofrontal contusion and expanding edema (A: day 1, B: day 10).

worsen after several days of delay. Not infrequently, these patients have been sent home and later develop refractory headache and become gradually more sleepy (Figure 3.2).

Most important is the development of displacement of brain tissues due to raised intracranial pressure or expanding intracranial mass lesions. Tissue may move into existing openings, which can lead to anatomical "herniation" under the falx, into the tentorial opening, or through the foramen magnum. With this displacement comes reduced cerebral perfusion, compression and buckling of surrounding tissues. Clinical signs are deepening of coma (motor responses changing to pathologic flexion or extension), new brainstem signs (changes in pupil size and eye motility), hypertension, tachypnea, and brady-cardia (Cushing reflex).

It is also known that TBI initiates a cascade of inflammatory processes and tissue damage up-regulates proinflammatory cytokines, chemokines, and endothelial-leukocyte adhesion molecules. There is release of glutamate and other excitatory amino acids, with influx of calcium into the cell resulting in characteristic apoptotic pathways that include the activation of caspases, free radical generation, and activation of calpains.[6,13,30] There is a significant excess of neurotransmitters that include glutamate, but also cholinergic excess that may enhance the destructive effects.[22] On the other hand, attempts to reduce cate-cholamine output by administering antagonists have a negative effect and reduce recovery from TBI.[15] Serotonergic pathways also may play a role and have been studied for possible pharmacotherapy. Most interesting is the recent discovery of a potential role of sex steroid hormones, with progesterone showing promise in mitigating the effects of excitotoxic injury.

A new pathway of research is the investigation of the role of microglia in traumatic head injury.[17] Microglia are cells of the brain that mediate response to infection in injury and belong to the mononuclear phagocyte lineage. Activated microglia may have a detrimental response due to induction of proinflammatory mediators that eventually contribute to reactive oxygen and nitrogen species. Microglia-related inflammation might become a study target.[25]

In Practice

It is useful to set certain rules for the recognition and management of TBI and what to be preoccupied with. There are decisions to be made immediately after admission and throughout the course of traumatic head injury.

JUDGING SEVERITY OF TRAUMATIC HEAD INJURY

There is one contentious issue—determining who needs a CT scan. Most patients, whether adult or children, will get a CT scan and may not need one.[21,49] There is very little compliance with current guidelines, and ordering of unnecessary CT scans continues.[37,45] Defensive medicine plays a role in the US healthcare system, driven by fear of missing a traumatic cerebral lesion or, even worse, missing a surgical lesion.[32] Over the years, several guidelines have been developed. The two best known are the New Orleans and Canadian CT scan rules. The New Orleans criteria[18,54] are highly sensitive and specific in identifying patients with what appears to be mild TBI but who have clinically important intracranial lesions, defined here as epidural hematoma, subdural hematoma, depressed skull fracture, cerebral contusion, or subarachnoid hemorrhage. In this model, seven variables are used: (1) presence of intoxication, (2) age >60 years, (3) prior seizure, (4) visible presence of trauma above the clavicles, (5) headache, (6) vomiting, and (7) short-term memory deficits. If all seven of these criteria are absent, the patient "does not really need" a CT scan of the brain. However, if one factor is present, the specificity is only 24%.

Another model is the Canadian CT rule, and the presenting Glasgow Coma Score (GCS) of 13–15 is an entry criteria. Five "high-risk" factors and two "medium-risk" factors are identified. The high-risk factors include (1) failure of the GCS to improve to reach its maximal score in 2 hours, (2) suspected open or depressed skull fracture, (3) two or more episodes of vomiting, (4) suspected basal skull fracture, and (5) age >65 years. The medium-risk factors are amnesia >30 minutes before the impact and a "dangerous mechanism" of injury.[54] The presence of any of the five high-risk factors has a specificity of 68%, and the presence of any of the seven criteria has a specificity of 49.6%. If applied, the Canadian Head CT scan rule may lead to a 20% decrease in the number of head CT scans and a 2.5-hour decrease in length of emergency department stay. However, several surveys have found that emergency room physicians either do not know the details of these models or do not apply them.[53,56] In a questionnaire, the common reasons for continuing to order a CT scan were to confirm or rule out a traumatic intracranial lesion and to expedite the diagnosis. "Fear of being sued" was a reason in 1 out of 5 answers, while "pressure from the patient or his relative" much less common (1 in 10). Unfortunately, these clinical decision rules did not prevent emergency physicians from ordering CT scans. An often-heard argument is that one CT scan with brief hospitalization can protect against a million-dollar lawsuit. Table 3.2 shows high-risk patients in need of a CT scan of the brain and likely other imaging studies.

Clinical decision rules in pediatrics are far more complicated.[31,36] The Pediatric Emergency Care Applied Research Network (PECARN) showed that using these rules, approximately 50 CT scans are needed to identify 1 child with clinically significant cranial injury, and more than 200 are necessary to identify neurosurgical injury.[24] The sensitivity of the PECARN rule was 0.99, and specificity was 0.54. Many studies have found that simply using level of consciousness or post-traumatic amnesia as entry criteria for CT scan could result in missing a significant number of patients who have TBI.[52]

INITIAL SUPPORT AFTER TRAUMATIC HEAD INJURY

The state of the airway and spine are the very first concerns. The first management in a patient with TBI is thus spinal precautions (placing a neck brace) and airway protection.[7,20,42] Securing an airway is a top priority. Patients are best intubated if level of consciousness is impaired and may include fiberoptic intubation. In massive soft tissue trauma, emergency tracheostomy may be needed, but often has

Table 3.2 **High-Risk Patients**

- Vehicle rollover
- Assault or fall
- Warfarin
- Antiplatelet agents
- Frontal contusions
- Fluid resuscitation with large amounts
---

already been performed in the field. Access to fluids needs to be secured with large bore IV catheter or, in some situations, intraosseous access. It is necessary to quickly obtain several physiologic parameters and normalize them (Table 3.3). Hypercapnia, hypoxemia, and hypotension are quite common in patients with severe TBI. These major systemic manifestations are often not immediately attended to,[26,39,59] but correction of these abnormalities is warranted.

If abnormalities are seen on the CT scan that could indicate increased intracranial pressure, an intracranial pressure (ICP) monitor can be placed, followed by adequate sedation and analgesia, usually a combination of propofol and fentanyl. This can then be followed by traditional methods of treatment of increased intracranial pressure with elevating the head of the bed 30 degrees and the use of hyperosmotic solutions such as mannitol and hypertonic saline.[3] Osmotic agents should be used if intracranial pressure is increased (or assumed to be increased) using 20% mannitol 1 g/kg or hypertonic saline 3% NaCl 30 mL IV over 5 minutes after a central access is assured. Some institutions have the opportunity to monitor brain oxygenation, but there is no established benefit of this information.[27,38] Temperature control is needed but early therapeutic hypothermia does not seem to impact on outcome. New trials to control ICP are planned.[1]

Fluid and blood pressure management is understandably important in the initial evaluation. Intravenous fluids are often used to maintain blood pressure; in hypotensive head injury patients, hypertonic saline improved cerebral perfusion pressure and increased brain oxygenation. Even administration of 250 mL 7.5% hypertonic saline after TBI improved outcome compared with 0.9 saline.[50]

THE MAJOR PRIORITIES IN TRAUMATIC BRAIN INJURY

Generally, there are eight major concerns early in the assessment and management of TBI. They should be systematically considered so as not to lose sight of the big picture, which can be befuddling at first.

Priority #1: Determine whether neurosurgical intervention is needed immediately. Neurologic examination ultimately matters, but decisions are also largely guided by the CT scan findings, and several CT scans may be necessary to more accurately judge an evolving contusion, epidural hematoma, or subdural hematoma.[48] There should be careful review of the CT scan that includes review of bone

Table 3.3 **Ideal Physiologic Values after TBI**

- Pulse oximetry >90%
- pH 7.35–7.45
- PaO_2 >100 mm Hg
- $PaCO_2$ 35–45 mm Hg
- Systolic blood pressure >90 mm Hg
- Intracranial pressure <20 mm Hg
- Cerebral perfusion pressure >60 mm Hg
- Temperature 36–38°C
- Glucose 140–180 mg/dL
- Na 135–140 mmol/L (145–160 mmol/L with hypertonic solutions)
- International normalized ratio <1.4
- Platelets >70.000
- Hgb >8 g/dL

Source: Data from reference 56.

windows for specific areas that can be affected. Fracture sites are associated with vascular injury, and this includes basal skull fracture and also fractures in the sphenoid sinus.

Management of penetrating injury is far more complicated, in particular when the injury traversed both hemispheres and when the diencephalic structures and mesencephalon are destroyed.[2,28] The presence of a hematoma on the CT scan, presence or absence of pupillary responses, and destruction of the diencephalon determine outcome. Neurosurgeons usually consider removal of bone and bullet fragments in patients with little or any involvement of level of consciousness.[43] Gunshots may also lacerate important arteries, such as the vertebral artery with gunshots through the oropharynx. In a matter of days, bullet fragments will eventually start to migrate due to cerebrospinal fluid pulsation.

Another important issue is the decision to proceed with evacuation of an acute epidural and subdural hematoma. The presence of an epidural hematoma on CT scan almost always indicates a neurosurgical indication. Outcome is determined by whether there is obliteration of the basal cisterns and whether there is a brain tissue shift of more than 5 mm, measured at the location of the septum pellucidum. Surgery for acute subdural hematoma is considered if the subdural hematoma has a thickness greater than 1 cm or midline shift of more than 5 mm on CT scan.[8] The decision to operate remains clear in some but arbitrary in others, but any patient with neurologic deterioration requires neurosurgical intervention. Surgery in large subdural hematomas with absence of many brainstem reflexes, particularly pupil and corneal, are likely not going to result in improved outcome. However, fixed pupils should not necessarily sway a neurosurgeon not to proceed with the evacuation.

Priority #2: Consider associated spinal cord injury and subsequently arrange to manage spinal cord injury. Full cervical spine X-rays and preferably a multiplanar CT are needed in any patient with TBI caused by a fall—even from standing height. Osteoligamentous injuries at the craniocervical junction are often associated with high-energy trauma. Odontoid fractures are easily missed and patients have a high risk of early and rapid clinical decline. In the early phase, realignment of displaced vertebra is necessary and requires a multidisciplinary response. Medical management includes early assessment of airway compromise, assessment for the presence of diaphragmatic dysfunction, and treatment of early autonomic dysreflexia (Chapter 4).

Priority #3: The patient may have multiorgan injury. Many centers use an injury severity score (ISS) that provides an overall score for patients with multiple injuries. Many of these injuries are not obvious and need close follow-up in the first 12–24 hours by a trauma surgeon even after the patient is admitted (Table 3.4).

Priority #4: The patient may be actively bleeding and would require reversal of an international normalized ratio (INR). Prothrombin complex, fresh frozen plasma, and vitamin K should be administered in any patient who has an INR greater than 2.0 or more than 1.5 if neurosurgical intervention is anticipated. In patients who need anticoagulation no progression on examination and stable contusion on CT scan 24–48 hours later may be considered for pharmacologic deep venous thrombosis prophylaxis.

Priority #5: The patient may need placement of an intracranial pressure monitoring device. Failure to aggressively control intracranial pressure to less than 20 mm Hg is common and particularly in the first hours, it could lead to early secondary brainstem injury. Decompressive surgery is an adequate treatment for increased intracranial pressure, and the threshold to proceed with this procedure

Table 3.4 **Injury Severity Score (ISS)**

Region	AIS
Head & Neck	1–6
Face	1–6
Chest	1–6
Abdomen	1–6
Extremities	1–6
External	1–6

The ISS is an anatomical scoring system that provides an overall score for patients with multiple injuries. Each injury is assigned an abbreviated injury scale (AIS) score and is allocated to one of six body regions (head, face, chest, abdomen, extremities [including pelvis], and external) (AIS score: 1 = minor, 2 = moderate, 3 = serious, 4 = severe, 5 = critical, 6 = not survivable). Only the highest AIS score in each body region is used. The three most severely injured body regions have their score squared and added together to produce the ISS score. With an injury and AIS of 6, ISS automatically defaults to 75.

should be generally low. Gunshot wounds to the head or blast injuries with contusions require immediate decompressive surgery. The outcome in these patients can be determined by a baseline neurologic examination. Fixed pupils in a comatose patient after a gunshot wound with hematoma involving both hemispheres indicates a poor outcome.[41]

Priority #6: Illicit drugs may confound the examination. Because TBI is often associated with intoxications, a blood and urinary toxicology screen and alcohol level should be obtained.

Priority #7: Consider foul play. In adults, TBI may be due to assault, which requires evaluation by the appropriate authorities. Any child with TBI may have been physically abused, which requires clinical recognition and early involvement of social or legal services.

Priority #8: Avoid early prognosticating or unnecessary pessimism. Many patients are young and have a tremendous resilience and may improve substantially. Neurologic examination may be deceiving early on. Nonetheless penetrating or blast injury remains very serious with high likelihood of very poor outcome.

By the Way

- Any severe TBI requires a repeat CT scan of the brain to detect contusions
- Alcohol intoxication in an established alcoholic rarely confounds neurologic examination
- Early hypotension associated with TBI is found in one out of three admissions and doubles the risk of mortality.
- Early hyperthermia increases length of intensive care unit stay, decreases recovery to a functional independence, and increases mortality
- Early hyperglycemia is common in TBI, but correction does not impact outcome

---

Traumatic Head Injury by the Numbers

- ~75% of TBI deteriorates from expanding hematoma
- ~60% of TBI is due to road traffic accidents
- ~50% of TBI and a skull fracture have an intracranial hematoma
- ~30% of TBI is due to falls, predominantly in the elderly
- ~20% of TBI may deteriorate after admission
- ~2% of TBI is caused by epidural hematoma

Putting It All Together

- TBI may require spine stabilization and a search for other traumatic injury
- TBI requires immediate neurosurgical intervention when there is penetrating trauma or mass effect
- TBI can appear mild but may result in rapid deterioration from new contusions
- TBI is highly unpredictable in the first days, so close follow-up is needed
- TBI requires transfer to a tertiary center if there is evidence of increased intra-cranial pressure or deterioration from brain tissue shift
- TBI requires specialized care in the emergency department

References

1. Andrews PJ, Sinclair LH, Harris B, et al. Study of therapeutic hypothermia (32 to 35°C) for intracranial pressure reduction after traumatic brain injury (the Eurotherm3235Trial): outcome of the pilot phase of the trial. *Trials* 2013;14:277.
2. Aryan HE, Jandial R, Bennett RL, et al. Gunshot wounds to the head: gang- and non-gang-related injuries and outcomes. *Brain Inj* 2005;19:505–510.
3. Baker AJ, Rhind SG, Morrison LJ, et al. Resuscitation with hypertonic saline-dextran reduces serum biomarker levels and correlates with outcome in severe traumatic brain injury patients. *J Neurotrauma* 2009;26:1227–1240.
4. Barrow A, Ndikum J, Harris T. Late presentations of minor head injury. *Emerg Med J* 2012;29:983–988.
5. Bigler ED. Anterior and middle cranial fossa in traumatic brain injury: Relevant neuroanatomy and neuropathology in the study of neuropsychological outcome, [review]. *Neuropsychology* 2007;21:515–531.
6. Block ML, Zecca L, Hong JS. Microglia-mediated neurotoxicity: uncovering the molecular mechanisms. *Nat Rev Neurosci* 2007;8:57–69.
7. Brain Trauma Foundation. Guidelines for the management of severe traumatic brain injury, 3rd ed. *J Neurotrauma* 2007;24:S1–S106.
8. Bullock MR, Chesnut R, Ghajar J, et al. Surgical management of acute subdural hematomas. *Neurosurgery* 2006;58:S16–S24.
9. Cohen DB, Rinker C, Wilberger JE. Traumatic brain injury in anticoagulated patients. *J Trauma* 2006;60:553–557.
10. Davis DP, Meade W, Sise MJ, et al. Both hypoxemia and extreme hyperoxemia may be detrimental in patients with severe traumatic brain injury. *J Neurotrauma* 2009;26:2217–2223.
11. DeKosky ST, Kochanek PM, Clark RS, Ciallella JR, Dixon CE. Secondary injury after head trauma: subacute and long-term mechanisms. *Semin Clin Neuropsychiatry* 1998;3:176–185.
12. DePalma RG, Burris DG, Champion HR., Hodgson MJ. Blast injuries. *N Engl J Med* 2005;352:1335–1342.
13. Farkas O, Povlishock JT. Cellular and subcellular change evoked by diffuse traumatic brain injury: a complex web of change extending far beyond focal damage. *Prog Brain Res* 2007;161:43–59.
14. Faul M, Xu L, Wald M, et al. *Traumatic Brain Injury in the United States: Emergency Department Visits, Hospitalizations, and Deaths 2002–2006.* Atlanta (GA), Centers for Disease Control and Prevention, National Center for Injury Prevention and Control, 2006.
15. Goldstein L. Neurotransmitters and motor activity: effects on functional recovery after brain injury. *NeuroRX* 2006;3:451–457.

16. Gönül E, Erdoğan E, Taşar M, et al. Penetrating orbitocranial gunshot injuries. *Surg Neurol* 2005;63:24–30.
17. Graeber MB, Streit WJ. Microglia: biology and pathology. *Acta Neuropathol* 2010;119:89–105.
18. Haydel MJ, Preston CA, Mills TJ, et al. Indications for computed tomography in patients with minor head injury. *N Engl J Med* 2000;343:100–105.
19. Hicks RR, Fertig SJ, Desrocher RE, Koroshetz WJ, Pancrazio JJ. Neurological effects of blast injury. *J Trauma* 2010;68:1257–1263.
20. Ingebrigtsen T, Romner B, Kock-Jensen C. Scandinavian guidelines for initial management of minimal, mild, and moderate head injuries. The Scandinavian Neurotrauma Committee. *J Trauma* 2000;48:760–766.
21. Jagoda AS, Bazarian JJ, Bruns JJ Jr, et al. Clinical policy: neuroimaging and decision making in adult mild traumatic brain injury in the acute setting. *Ann Emerg Med* 2008;52:714–748.
22. Johnson VE, Stewart W, Smith DH. Axonal pathology in traumatic brain injury. *Exp Neurol* 2012 Jan 20. [Epub ahead of print]
23. Kolias AG, Guilfoyle MR, Helmy A, et al. Traumatic brain injury in adults. *Pract Neurol* 2013;13:228–235.
24. Kuppermann N, Holmes JF, Dayan PS, et al. Identification of children at very low risk of clinically-important brain injuries after head trauma: a prospective cohort study. *Lancet* 2009;374:1160–1170.
25. Loane DJ, Byrnes KR. Role of microglia in neurotrauma. *Neurotherapeutics* 2010;7:366–377.
26. Manley G, Knudson MM, Morabito D, Damron S, Erickson V, Pitts L. Hypotension, hypoxia, and head injury: frequency, duration, and consequences. *Arch Surg* 2001;136:1118–1123.
27. Martini RP, Deem S, Treggiari MM. Targeting brain tissue oxygenation in traumatic brain injury. *Resp Care* 2013;58:162–167.
28. Martins RS, Siqueira MG, Santos MT, Zanon-Collange N, Moraes OJ. Prognostic factors and treatment of penetrating gunshot wounds to the head. *Surg Neurol* 2003;60:98–104.
29. McAllister TW. Neurobiological consequences of traumatic brain injury. *Dialogues Clin Neurosci* 2011;13:287–300.
30. McIntosh TK, Smith DH, Meaney DF, et al. Neuropathological sequelae of traumatic brain injury: relationship to neurochemical and biomechanical mechanisms. *Lab Invest* 1996;74:315–342.
31. Medwid K, Couri GG. How accurate are clinical decision rules for pediatric minor head injury? *Ann Emerg Med* 2012;68:278–279.
32. Mello MM, Chandra A, Gawande AA, Studdert DM. National costs of the medical liability system. *Health Aff (Millwood)* 2010;29:1569–1577.
33. Menon D., Schwab K., Wright D., Maas A. Position statement: definition of traumatic brain injury. *Arch Phys Med Rehabil* 2010;91:1637–1640.
34. Meythaler J., Peduzzi J., Eleftheriou E., et al. Current concepts: diffuse axonal injury associated traumatic brain injury. *Arch Phys Med Rehabil* 2001;82:1461–1471.
35. Misra J., Chakravart S. A study of rotational brain injury. *J Biomech* 1984;17:459–466.
36. Morton MJ, Korley FK. Head computed tomography use in the emergency department for mild traumatic brain injury: integrating evidence into practice for the resident physician. *Ann Emerg Med.* 2012;60:361–367.
37. Mower WR, Hoffman JR, Herbert M, et al. Developing a clinical decision instrument to rule out intracranial injuries in patients with minor head trauma: methodology of the NEXUS II investigation. *Ann Emerg Med* 2002;40:505–514.
38. Narotam PK, Morrison JF, Nathoo N. Brain tissue oxygen monitoring in traumatic brain injury and major trauma: outcome analysis of a brain tissue oxygen-directed therapy. *J Neurosurg* 2009;111:672–682.
39. Pascual JL, Maloney-Wilensky E, Reilly PM, et al. Resuscitation of hypotensive head-injured patients: is hypertonic saline the answer? *Am Surg* 2008;74:253–259.
40. Peterson EC, Chesnut RM. Talk and die revisited: bifrontal contusions and late deterioration. *J Trauma* 2011;71:1588–1592.

41. Polin RS, Shaffrey ME, Phillips CD, Germanson T, Jane JA. Multivariate analysis and prediction of outcome following penetrating head injury. *Neurosurg Clin N Am* 1995;6:689–699.

42. Protheroe RT, Gwinnutt CL. Early hospital care of severe traumatic brain injury. *Anaesthesia* 2011;66:1035–1047.

43. Ragel BT, Klimo P Jr, Martin JE, et al. Wartime decompressive craniectomy: technique and lessons learned. *Neurosurg Focus* 2010;28:E2.

44. Reilly PL. Brain injury: the pathophysiology of the first hours; "Talk and Die revisited." *J Clin Neurosci* 2001;8:398–403.

45. Rohacek M, Albrecht M, Kleim B, Zimmermann H, Exadaktylos A. Reasons for ordering computed tomography scans of the head in patients with minor brain injury. *Injury* 2012 Jan 23. [Epub ahead of print]

46. Rutland-Brown W, Langlois JA., Thomas KE, Xi YL. Incidence of traumatic brain injury in the United States, 2003. *J Head Trauma Rehabil* 2006;21:544–548.

47. Sabet A., Christoforou E., Zatlin B., et al. Deformation of the human brain induced by mild angular head acceleration. *J Biomech* 2008;41:307–315.

48. Servadei F, Nasi MT, Giuliani G, et al. CT prognostic factors in acute subdural haematomas: the value of the "worst" CT scan. *Br J Neurosurg* 2000;14:110–116.

49. Servadei F, Teasdale G, Merry G. Defining acute mild head injury in adults: a proposal based on prognostic factors, diagnosis, and management. *J Neurotrauma* 2001;18:657–664.

50. Shackford SR, Bourguignon PR, Wald SL, Rogers FB, Osler TM, Clark DE. Hypertonic saline resuscitation of patients with head injury: a prospective, randomized clinical trial. *J Trauma* 1998;44:50–58.

51. Shahlaie K, Keachie K, Hutchins IM, et al. Risk factors for posttraumatic vasospasm. *J Neurosurg* 2011;115:602–611.

52. Sheehan A, Batchelor JS. A retrospective cohort study to re-evaluate clinical correlates for intracranial injury in minor head injury. *Emerg Med J.* 2011;29:899–901.

53. Stiell IG, Clement CM, Rowe BH, et al. Comparison of the Canadian CT Head Rule and the New Orleans Criteria in patients with minor head injury. *JAMA* 2005;294:1511–1518.

54. Stiell IG, Wells GA, Vandemheen K, et al. The Canadian CT Head Rule for patients with minor head injury. *Lancet* 2001;357:1391–1396.

55. Strich SJ. Shearing of nerve fibres as a cause of brain damage due to head injury: a pathological study of twenty cases. *Lancet* 1961;278:443–448.

56. Swadron S, LeRoux P, Smith W, Weingart SD. Emergency neurological life support: traumatic brain injury. *Neurocrit Care* 2012 17 Supl 1: S112–121.

57. Swartz KR, Fee DB, Dempsey RJ. Blossoming traumatic epidural hematoma. *J Emerg Med* 2003;25:451–452.

58. Tauber M, Koller H, Moroder P, Hitzl W, Resch H. Secondary intracranial hemorrhage after mild head injury in patients with low-dose acetylsalicylate acid prophylaxis. *J Trauma* 2009;67:521–525.

59. Trivedi M, Coles JP. Blood pressure management in acute head injury. *J Intensive Care Med* 2009;24:96–107.

4

Recognition of Acute Spinal Cord Injury

Acute spinal cord injury is frequently due to spinal cord compression and may present with easily identifiable signs (inability to stand or walk) or, conversely, be very difficult to detect (fever and back pain in epidural abscess). Spinal cord compression is considerably better imaged with the availability of MRI of the spine. Such MRI scans are able to not only detect compression but also identify intrinsic cord lesions and abnormal vasculature. The reality, however, is that the availability of MRI is limited—particularly after hours—but it is still more common that physicians fail to recognize an acute spinal cord injury's signs and symptoms.[17,18] It is expected that a neurologist and neurosurgeon can quickly recognize spinal cord compression. A good knowledge of the neuroanatomy and specific syndromes is needed.

Acute spinal cord injury may be traumatic or nontraumatic, and its management involves mostly neurosurgeons or spine surgeons. This area of neurology is prone to misjudgments, errors, and complications, mostly as a result of ambiguous presentation by the patient. Most hyperacute myeloradiculopathies, defined as emerging within minutes or hours, are either traumatic or vascular in origin. Spinal cord compression usually takes days or weeks, although a sudden worsening may occur.[5,6,15,22,30] The damage done by acute spinal cord compression is substantial and often permanent.[34,41] Myelopathies due to less common causes such as inflammatory or heredodegenerative disorders are usually chronic.

So where are the priorities? When should we press on for immediate diagnostic tests? What are the difficulties with pinpointing a cause? How can we prevent further harm? This chapter briefly touches on mechanisms and discusses clinical assessment and treatment in detail.

Principles

INJURY MECHANISMS

Some words on injury mechanisms are needed. The biochemistry of acute spinal cord injury is not entirely understood but involves rapid destruction of neuronal networks. What has been recognized is that in the spinal cord there are multiple inhibitory factors for axonal regeneration. As opposed to the peripheral nervous system, the central nervous system has very limited regeneration of severed fibers.[10] Regeneration, if any, is extremely protracted, and there is a paucity of expression of growth factors. It is assumed that the glial scar that occurs within days of injury inhibits axonal regeneration and contains growth inhibitory molecules. In addition, long-distance axonal regeneration does not occur[24,47] (Figure 4.1). Furthermore, the upper motor neurons have no cell-intrinsic growth programs and no formation of bridges by Schwann cells. Macrophages or fibroblasts do appear, making regeneration virtually impossible.

Molecular signals associated with axonal growth have been identified, and regeneration-associated genes are upregulated. Therapeutic approaches may focus on improving axonal sprouting, but clinical trials were not successful in improving clinical outcome. Examples are minocycline (inhibitor of excitotoxicity), cyclosporin (immunosuppression), and erythropoietin (neuroprotection and preventing apoptosis).

In addition, there might be vascular mechanisms. Initially there might be an ischemic insult to the spinal cord that then may be further damaged in a phase of hyperemia, causing cord reperfusion with inflammatory mediators. During this reperfusion there is increased glutamate and aspartate in the CSF, all contributing to further injury.

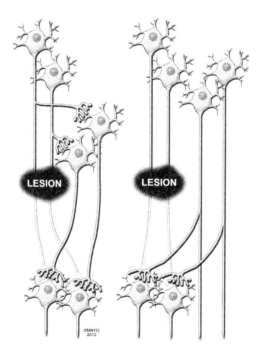

Figure 4.1 Sprouting after acute spinal cord injury.

There is active research in cell-mediated therapy that includes intrathecal injection of bone marrow–derived cells or intraparenchymal injection of Schwann cells. Benefits have not yet been demonstrated, and the high incidence of additional neuropathic pain after such a treatment—possibly indicating new neuronal circuitry—requires more study.[14]

NEUROLOGIC LOCALIZATION

First, there are useful localization principles. There is a reasonable consistency to the organization of long tracts.[11] There are several immediate cues that would indicate a compression of the spinal cord from a nearby space occupying tumor or hematoma. Patients have weakness below the level of the lesion, often with upper motor neuron and lower motor neuron signs, abnormal sphincter function, and sensory loss involving all modalities. The sacral dermatomas are involved, because the fibers of the spinothalamic tracts lie close to the surface of the cord and are the first to become compressed.

If a sensory level is found, it indicates the level of the compression but it may involve several segments above the lesion. This is important, because an MRI of the spine may typically involve a narrow view of segments of the spinal cord and other segments can be easily missed if not fully imaged (e.g., lumbar MRI will not image the majority of the thoracic spine). Therefore, any patient with spinal cord compression should have an MRI of the entire spine to avoid missing a surgically treatable lesion. Failing to image the lesion, placing too much emphasis on the sensory level alone, may lead to a missed opportunity.

Several cord syndromes have been described. A central cord syndrome, in which patients have damage to the central gray matter but sparing of the long tracts, features more conspicuous lower motor neuron signs in the upper extremities without long tract features. The sacral dermatoma are spared as is the anal reflex. It is typically seen in intramedullary spinal tumors or after traumatic spine injury. Anterior cord syndrome results in paraplegia or tetraplegia, absent pain and temperature sensation below the lesion, but sparing of the dorsal column function, with intact vibration and position sense. A hemicord syndrome is diagnosed with corticospinal tract and dorsal column function abnormal on one side but abnormal pain and temperature sensation on the opposite side, and is indicative of trauma or a compressive cord lesion. The most commonly missed diagnosis is the acute cauda equina syndrome, in which the weakness of the lower limbs is mild but there is profound sphincter abnormality and subtle anesthesia. The presence of bilateral leg pain is also an important cue. This is typically seen from compression of the cord and cauda equina due to an extradural tumor or central disc prolapse. The outcome can be generally predicted based on whether the patient can walk at presentation—and is potentially good—although long-term improvement has been described in patients with severe spinal cord involvement.[21,39]

There are several other major core principles in neurologic examinations to discuss. In sensory examination pin sharpness should be recognized and, if absent, it should be considered abnormal (comparison with facial pin prick is useful). There are easy-to-remember landmarks with the nipple at T4, navel at T10, and midway arm to chest on the C4-T2 border. Because the T3 and C4 dermatoma may vary and overlap, mistakes are made here. Sensory examinations of the genital and rectal area are exceedingly important but often not performed in great detail or totally avoided. Important tests may include the anal wink (a safety-pin poking resulting in anal contraction) and the much less frequently performed bulbocavernosus reflex (gloved finger in the rectum with pull at Foley catheter or squeezing the head of the penis).

Motor examination should include 20 muscles (the so-called key muscles) and should differentiate between voluntary and involuntary movements (spasms may be common). Palpation of muscles may be needed to detect contraction. Several muscles point toward the region of abnormalities: deltoid and biceps for C5, brachioradialis and extensor carpi radialis longus for C6, triceps for C7, wrist and finger flexors for C8, intrinsic muscles of the hand for T1, quadriceps for L3, quadriceps and tibialis anterior for T4, extensor hallucis longus for L5, and gastrocnemius for S1. Combination of these abnormalities could also help in determining the abnormality of the lesion.

The abnormalities are best categorized into complete or incomplete status and summarized in an ASIA scale (Table 4.1). ASIA grade A in traumatic injury indicates a low probability of recovery, with less than 5% improving to functional strength.[20] Incomplete paraplegia levels increase the change of mobility greatly—up to two-thirds of the patients.

Another useful designation is to use the N-O-O-O-O-N sign. The first N stands for voluntary anal contraction, the Os for light touch left and right and pin prick

Table 4.1 **ASIA Impairment Grading for Spinal Cord Injury**

A	Complete	No motor or sensory function preserved in sacral (S4-S5) segments
B	Incomplete	Sensory but not motor function preserved below level including sacral (S4-S5) levels
C	Incomplete	Motor function preserved below level (more than half of key muscles and >MRC of 3)
E	Incomplete	Motor and sensory function normal

Proceed as follows:
• Determine sensory level (most caudal)
• Determine motor level (lowest key muscle of MRC ≥3)
• Determine complete or incomplete
• Designate as: central cord, Brown-Séquard, anterior cord, conus medullaris, cauda equina

ASIA: American spinal injury association.

Table 4.2 **Causes of Myelopathy**

Cause	Extrinsic	Intrinsic
Traumatic	Vertebral fracture or dislocation	Missile or stab injuries
Infective	Epidural abscess Tuberculous osteomyelitis	Acute viral myelitis Tuberculosis Syphilis Schistosomiasis HIV HTLV-1
Inflammatory	Rheumatoid arthritis Ankylosing spondylitis	Multiple sclerosis Neuromyelitis optica Sarcoidosis, Behçet Connective tissue disorders
Neoplastic	Extradural tumors Extramedullary- intradural tumors	Intramedullary tumors Paraneoplastic
Vascular	Epidural hematoma Dural arteriovenous fistula	Hematomyelia Ischemic infarction
Metabolic	Paget's disease	Vitamin B_{12} deficiency Copper deficiency Liver failure
Toxic	Intrathecal MTX	Cisplatin Nitrous oxide Clioquinol Lathyrism, Konzo
Degenerative	Spondylosis Disc prolapse	Amyotrophic lateral sclerosis Primary lateral sclerosis

Source: Modified from reference 11.
HIV: human immunodeficiency virus; HTLV-1: human T-lymphotropic virus-1; MTX: methotrexate

left and right, and the last N stands for absent anal sensation. Presence of the N-O-O-O-O-N sign signifies a complete injury.

Next, causes need to be considered. It is practically useful to separate acute spinal cord compression into traumatic versus nontraumatic and nontraumatic into cancer-related and other causes. A long list of causes of myelopathies are shown in Table 4.2 but many are very uncommon.[1] These can be investigated by performing a spinal fluid examination that should include cells, protein, oligoclonal bands, and specific PCRs. It should also include an autoimmune panel as well as HIV and HTLV-1 serology to assist in the diagnosis.

In Practice

Acute traumatic spinal cord injury involves the cervical cord in 50% of the cases, with 35% in a thoracic segment. Complete cord lesions are much less prevalent due to improved care in the field and increased use of seat belts but, nonetheless, still may occur on a regular basis. After initial stabilization, medical and surgical care of acute spinal cord injury requires attention focused on examination and immediate assessment of risks. Details of surgical management are not discussed here and are in the hands of a trauma surgeon or neurosurgeon. However, the neurologist can play an important role not only in localizing the lesion but also in providing early supportive medical care. Immediate urinary catheter placement, gastric ulcer prophylaxis, correction of core hypothermia, and deep venous thrombosis prophylaxis are pertinent. Volume resuscitation or vasopressors are is often initially needed to correct hypotension.

Studies have looked at ways to better standardize assessment and the best known are the NEXUS criteria (found at www.medcalc.com). The mnemonic is NSAID, with N for neurologic deficit, S for midline spinal tenderness, A for altered consciousness, I for intoxication, and D for distracting injury. Distracting injury applies to long bone fracture, large burns, visceral injury, crush injury, and any other injury focusing attention away from spinal cord injury. Only if these criteria are absent can the spine be cleared clinically with a plain X-ray. Despite these criteria, it is likely that patients with a strong suspicion of spine injury will undergo a full CT scan. Such a CT scan study should be multiplanar. Spine instability is probable if not certain when there is a widened spinal space or fascia joints, anterolisthesis, and narrowed or widened disk space. These abnormalities can be easily detected on MRI scan of the spine.

ACUTE MANAGEMENT OF TRAUMATIC SPINE INJURY

Acute medical management of traumatic spine injury involves a combination of commonsensical measures followed by more specialized treatment. Outcome may be much worse if acute changes in respiratory function, autonomic failure and abnormal peristalsis are not managed acutely.

The interval between trauma and examination is important because, within the first three hours, methylprednisolone 30 mg/kg can be administered followed by infusion of 5.5 mg/kg hourly for 24 hours. If the patient is seen in the interval between three to eight hours, the infusion of methylprednisolone is continued for 48 hours but with a similar bolus of 30 mg/kg. This practice of using IV methyl prednisolone is variable (due to concerns with prior clinical trials), less frequent then years ago and some neurosurgens do simply not use it.

Surgical intervention after traumatic spinal cord trauma is typically performed to improve early surgical stabilization. There are some who advocate for early surgical stabilization and others who prefer late surgical stabilization (defined as greater than 72 hours after trauma) for optimal patient outcome (Figure 4.2). The current data show that patients who received early surgical stabilization had shorter hospital intensive care unit (ICU) stays, fewer days on the ventilator, and thus fewer pulmonary complications.[36]

Immobilization of the cervical spine is usually performed by emergency medical services and should involve the use of Philadelphia or Miami J collars. Management of traumatic spine injury often involves immediate closed reduction and surgical realignment.[7,8,9,12,28,45] A patient is often placed in a halo fixator followed by later instrumentation and stabilization. Anterior decompression is strongly considered by spine trauma surgeons if there is still residual anterior compression after realignment.

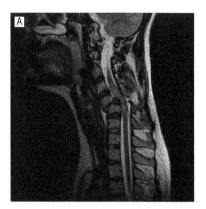
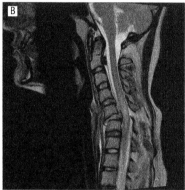
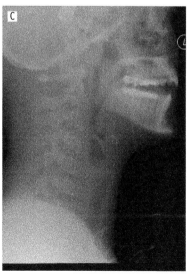

Figure 4.2 Closed reduction of a C5–C6 fracture: A: C5–C6 dislocation; B: C5–C6 dislocation post reduction; C: reduced C5–C6 dislocation.

A immediate medical stabilization may be needed, which includes endotracheal intubation in patients with respiratory difficulties. Patients may be in obvious respiratory distress, barely maintaining oxygen saturation, and there may be use of accessory muscles, inability to hold breath for 10 seconds, and abdominal paradox (outward abdominal movement with inspiration in a rocking-horse motion).

Respiratory compromise can be detected using pulmonary function tests which pinpoint diaphragmatic involvement. Usually involvement of C5-C6 musculature will make it likely that the respiration parameters may decline rapidly. Respiratory compromise may also be due to the rapid development of atelectasis and mucus plugs. For that reason, the patient should be immediately placed in a rotary bed, while use of the incentive spirometer at regular intervals is encouraged. Pattern of breathing in tetraplegia is typically small tidal volumes, increased respiratory rate, but no major change in minute ventilation. Early respiratory complications are rapidly developing atelectasis and pneumonia, occurring in over 50% of patients with the prevalence increasing with the time in the ICU. When patients undergo anterior cervical spine surgery, regional edema may considerably compromise airway, in particular if three or four cervical levels are exposed. In many patients, prolonged intubation (1 to 2 days) after surgery may be needed. Many patients with C2–C3 level injury will recover diaphragmatic function, and weaning can start with vital capacity of 15 mL/kg.

After a major injury, the circulation is immediately at risk due to loss of sympathetic tone. Hypotension from unopposed parasympathetic tone is very common, resulting in shock from vasodilatation. The typical finding is warm extremities but marked hypotension from redistribution to the peripheral circulation. It is prudent to place a central venous catheter (internal jugular or peripherally inserted central catheter) and to start norepinephrine infusion immediately to maintain adequate tissue perfusion. It is recommended to maintain a mean arterial pressure of 85 mmHg for 7 days. Hemodynamic instability is also a later concern. Hypotension is worsened by rapid position change, dehydration, and early sepsis as well as by medications such as narcotics, diuretics, and antidepressants. Midodrine or fludrocortisone is useful.

Autonomic dysreflexia may be seen early with cord lesions at the T6 level or higher. Bladder extension or bowel distension may trigger unopposed sympathetic activity resulting in hypertension, pounding headaches, skin flushing above the sensory thoracic level, goose bumps, bradycardia, and anxiety. Treatment involves finding the cause, improve catheter drainage, to relieve fecal impaction, and may require brief use of intravenous antihypertensives.

Bowel perforation may have occurred and may not be sensed by the patient. The diagnosis (or clinical signs for that matter) can be missed if physicians are simply not aware of the possibility. Abdominal X-rays or CT scan are needed to monitor the development and guide treatment. Virtually all patients in the acute spinal shock phase have no bowel sounds. A rectal suppository can be used, but an adynamic ileus can be anticipated for several days. Colace, Senokot, and rectal suppositories may be useful initially. All patients have a neurogenic bladder that requires urinary catheter placement.

The skin should be immediately looked at and is compromised. Gel pads might be necessary to relieve pain and compression, particularly in patients who are in cervical traction. Patients should be treated with subcutaneous heparin unless spine instrumentation is anticipated in the next 48 hours. In the long term, most likely an inferior vena cava filter will have to be placed to prevent fatal pulmonary emboli; but this procedure in patients with cervical or thoracic cord lesions is controversial, and there is insufficient data using these filter devices preemptively. Aggressive early pain management with codeine and anxiolytic medications is often required. Pain is an early concerning symptom but is usually provoked due to declined pain threshold (hyperalgesia). Long-term pain relief options other than pharmacotherapeutic options (antidepressants, anticonvulsants, or opioids) tend to be less effective. Painful muscle spasms (often burning hot) come later and are very difficult to control medically, often requiring Baclofen pumps.

ACUTE MANAGEMENT OF SPINAL CORD COMPRESSION

Another management problem is acute spinal cord compression.[2,3,26,43] Nontraumatic spinal cord compression often is due to malignant spinal cord compression and is more common in terminally ill cancer patients, with a median survival less than six months.[38,46] Much of the malignant spinal cord compression is in the epidural space and likely originates from vertebrae or impingement via neural foramina. Cancers that most likely cause acute spinal cord compression are lung, breast, and prostate, multiple myeloma, non-Hodgkin lymphoma, and renal cell carcinoma.[40] It has been found that breast and lung cancer more often metastasize to the thoracic spine, while abdominal and lung cancer metastasize more commonly to the lumbosacral area.

The diagnosis of spinal cord compression is considered clinically and is followed by an MRI that further delineates the abnormality. MRI should include a T1- and T2-weighted image in the axial-sagittal and coronal planes. Often metastases have multiple localizations.

The treatment is immediate administration of IV corticosteroids.[25] A bolus of 10 mg dexamethasone is administered followed by 16 mg per day, usually in a twice-daily or four-times-daily dose to improve tolerance. Ambulatory status remains the most important prognosticating factor. When patients are not ambulant and have a dense paresis, a much higher dexamethasone dose of 100 mg can be considered with variable maintenance dose of 16–96 mg over 5 days.[13, 42,44] Usually surgeons use minimally invasive techniques, which should be considered in patients who have a good prognosis and are medically operable. Radiotherapy is indicated in patients with a poor prognosis. In general, radiotherapy is usually a preferred treatment in patients with metastatic epidural spinal cord compression.[16,19,21,32,33,35,37,43] However, there are selective situations when surgery is indicated before radiotherapy. Radiosensitive tumors include lymphoma, myeloma, breast, prostate, and small cell lung cancers. Radioresistant tumors include melanoma, sarcoma, and renal cell carcinomas. Indications for radiation alone include prior radical spinal decompression, stable finding with no clinical evidence of cord compression, or most often the patient being a poor surgical candidate, usually patients with an anticipated survival of less than three months. Chemotherapy may only have a role in the primary treatment of spinal cord compression due to lymphoma, plasma cell tumor, and germ cell tumor, or previously untreated small cell carcinoma of the lung.

Prognosis can be determined by the Maranzano criteria and this may guide the decision to proceed with surgery. Accepted indications for surgery are displacement with bony impingement of the spinal cord, worsening of symptoms during or soon after spinal radiotherapy, paralysis of rapid onset, high cervical spine involvement, and no previous histological diagnosis of malignancy.

Surgery can still be indicated in a patient with a spinal instability as defined by a bony retropulsion into the canal, the presence of pathological fractures prior radiation therapy to the area, known radioresistant tumor paraplegia for less than 48 hours; and a restricted area of cord compression.[4,27,29,31]

Less common causes for spinal cord compression are epidural abscess and epidural hematoma. Recognition of an epidural abscess is notoriously difficult because the presentation can be very similar to pyelonephritis and cholecystitis. The physician should be alert to the diagnosis in an acutely febrile patient without an obvious source of infection and with rapidly developing weakness or a cord syndrome. Emergency drainage after surgical exploration is followed by antibiotic therapy for 8 weeks. Spinal epidural hematomas are equally uncommon but usually expected in patients who are anticoagulated. Immediate reversal of anticoagulation and evacuation within 12 hours results in good ambulatory function and bladder control.

Putting It All Together

- ASIA impairment assessment is key to determine management and to prognosticate
- The N-O-O-O-O-N sign determines complete lesion
- Circulation is best supported with vasopressors aiming at a mean arterial pressure of 85 mm Hg
- Respiratory compromise can be expected if C5-C6 innervated muscles are weak
- NEXUS criteria may help in determining spine instability after trauma
- Surgery for cancer-associated spine compression is indicated with rapid worsening of symptoms or if there is any impingement of the cord
- Radiotherapy is the first-line approach in most patients with metastatic epidural spinal cord compression

---

By the Way

- Cervical spine clearance in stuporous patients requires MRI
- Urgent decompression after spinal cord injury is indicated in patients with neurologic deterioration
- Autonomic dysreflexia may be due to inadequate bladder drainage
- Sympathetic denervations (T1-L3 level) may eliminate the febrile response and mask infection

---

Acute Spinal Cord Injury by the Numbers

- ~90% with complete TSCI develop dysautonomia
- ~60% with TSCI lesion below C4 can be weaned from the ventilator
- ~50% with complete TSCI but sacral sparing improve motor function
- ~50% with surgery for spinal cord compression become ambulant
- ~20% have normal bladder with late epidural hematoma removal

References

1. Brinar VV, Habek M, Brinar M, Malojčić B, Boban M. The differential diagnosis of acute transverse myelitis. *Clin Neurol Neurosurg* 2006;108:278–283.
2. Cavaliere R, Schiff D. Epidural spinal cord compression. *Curr Treat Options Neurol* 2004;6:285–295.
3. Chaichana KL, Woodworth GF, Sciubba DM, et al. Predictors of ambulatory function after decompressive surgery for metastatic epidural spinal cord compression. *Neurosurgery* 2008;62:683–692.
4. Chen YJ, Chang GC, Chen HT, et al. Surgical results of metastatic spinal cord compression secondary to non-small cell lung cancer. *Spine* 2007;32:E413–E418.
5. Cole JS, Patchell RA. Metastatic epidural spinal cord compression. *Lancet Neurol* 2008;7:459–466.
6. Copeman MC. Presenting symptoms of neoplastic spinal cord compression. *J Surg Oncol* 1988;37:24–25
7. Dimar JR, Carreon LY, Riina J, Schwartz DG, Harris MB. Early versus late stabilization of the spine in the polytrauma patient. *Spine* 2010;35:S187–S192.
8. Fehlings MG, Wilson JR. Timing of surgical intervention in spinal trauma: what does the evidence indicate? *Spine* 2010;35:S159–S160.
9. Furlan JC, Noonan V, Cadotte DW, Fehlings MG. Timing of decompressive surgery of spinal cord after traumatic spinal cord injury: an evidence-based examination of pre-clinical and clinical studies. *J Neurotrauma* 2011;28:1371–1399.
10. Giger RJ, Hollis ER 2nd, Tuszynski MH. Guidance molecules in axon regeneration. *Cold Spring Harb Perspect Biol* 2010;2:a001867.
11. Ginsberg L. Disorders of the spinal cord and roots. *Pract Neurol* 2011;11:259–267.
12. Gore PA, Chang S, Theodore N. Cervical spine injuries in children: attention to radiographic differences and stability compared to those in the adult patient. *Semin Pediatr Neurol* 2009;16:42–58.

13. Graham PH, Capp A, Delaney G, et al. A pilot randomized comparison of dexamethasone 96 mg vs 16 mg per day for malignant spinal-cord compression treated by radiotherapy: TROG 01.05 Superdex study. *Clin Oncol (R Coll Radiol)* 2006;18:70–76.

14. Harrop JS, Hashimoto R, Norvell D, et al. Evaluation of clinical experience using cell-based therapies in patients with spinal cord injury: a systematic review. *J Neurosurg Spine* 2012;17:230–246.

15. Helweg-Larsen S, Sørensen PS. Symptoms and signs in metastatic spinal cord compression: a study of progression from first symptom until diagnosis in 153 patients. *Eur J Cancer* 1994;30A:396–398.

16. Holt T, Hoskin P, Maranzano E, et al. Malignant epidural spinal cord compression: the role of external beam radiotherapy. *Curr Opin Support Palliat Care* 2012;6:103–108.

17. Husband DJ, Grant KA, Romaniuk CS. MRI in the diagnosis and treatment of suspected malignant spinal cord compression. *Br J Radiol* 2001;74:15–23.

18. Kim JK, Learch TJ, Colletti PM, et al. Diagnosis of vertebral metastasis, epidural metastasis, and malignant spinal cord compression: are T(1)-weighted sagittal images sufficient? *Magn Reson Imaging* 2000;18:819–824.

19. Klimo P Jr, Thompson CJ, Kestle JR, Schmidt MH. A meta-analysis of surgery versus conventional radiotherapy for the treatment of metastatic spinal epidural disease. *Neuro Oncol* 2005;7:64–76.

20. Kirshblum S, Millis S, McKinley W, Tulsky D. Late neurologic recovery after traumatic spinal cord injury. *Arch Phys Med Rehab* 2004;85:1811–1817.

21. Krishna V, Andrews HK, Varma A, et al. Spinal cord injury: How can we improve the classification and quantification of its severity and prognosis? *J Neurotrauma.* 2013;Jul 29. [Epub ahead of print]

22. Loblaw DA, Mitera G, Ford M, Laperriere NJ. A 2011 updated systematic review and clinical practice guideline for the management of malignant extradural spinal cord compression. *Int J Radiat Oncol Biol Phys* 2012;84:312–317.

23. Loblaw DA, Perry J, Chambers A, Laperriere NJ. Systematic review of the diagnosis and management of malignant extradural spinal cord compression: the Cancer Care Ontario Practice Guidelines Initiative's Neuro-Oncology Disease Site Group. *Clin Oncol* 2005;23:2028–2037.

24. Lu P, Jones LL, Tuszynski MH. Axon regeneration through scars and into sites of chronic spinal cord injury. *Exp Neurol* 2007;203:8–21.

25. McCurdy MT, Shanholtz CB. Oncologic emergencies. *Crit Care Med* 2012;40:2212–2222.

26. National Collaborating Centre for Cancer. *Metastatic Spinal Cord Compression: Diagnosis and Management of Patients at Risk of or with Metastatic Spinal Cord Compression.* Cardiff, Author, 2008.

27. North RB, LaRocca VR, Schwartz J, et al. Surgical management of spinal metastases: analysis of prognostic factors during a 10-year experience. *J Neurosurg Spine* 2005;2:564–573.

28. Oner FC, Wood KB, Smith JS, Shaffrey CI. Therapeutic decision making in thoracolumbar spine trauma. *Spine (Phila Pa 1976)* 2010;35:S235–S244.

29. Patchell RA, Tibbs PA, Regine WF, et al. Direct decompressive surgical resection in the treatment of spinal cord compression caused by metastatic cancer: a randomized trial. *Lancet* 2005;366:643–648.

30. Prasad D, Schiff D. Malignant spinal-cord compression. *Lancet Oncol* 2005;6:15–24.

31. Prewett S, Venkitaraman R. Metastatic spinal cord compression: review of the evidence for a radiotherapy dose fractionation schedule. *Clin Oncol (R Coll Radiol)* 2010;22:222–230.

32. Rades D, Abrahm JL. The role of radiotherapy for metastatic epidural spinal cord compression. *Nat Rev Clin Oncol* 2010;7:590–598.

33. Rades D, Blach M, Bremer M, et al. Prognostic significance of the time of developing motor deficits before radiation therapy in metastatic spinal cord compression: one-year results of a prospective trial. *Int J Radiat Oncol Biol Phys* 2000;48:1403–1408.

34. Rades D, Douglas S, Veninga T, et al. Metastatic spinal cord compression in non-small cell lung cancer patients. Prognostic factors in a series of 356 patients. *Strahlenther Onkol* 2012;188:472–476.

35. Rades D, Douglas S, Veninga T, et al. Prognostic factors in a series of 504 breast cancer patients with metastatic spinal cord compression. *Strahlenther Onkol* 2012;188:340–345.
36. Rades D, Dunst J, Schild SE. The first score predicting overall survival in patients with metastatic spinal cord compression. *Cancer* 2008;112:157–161.
37. Rades D, Stalpers LJ, Veninga T, et al. Evaluation of five radiation schedules and prognostic factors for metastatic spinal cord compression. *J Clin Oncol* 2005;23:3366–3375.
38. Ribas ES, Schiff D. Spinal cord compression. *Curr Treat Options Neurol* 2012;14: 391–401.
39. Robertson CE, Brown RD Jr, Wijdicks EFM, Rabinstein AA. Recovery after spinal cord infarcts: long-term outcome in 115 patients. *Neurology* 2012;78:114–121.
40. Schiff D, Batchelor T, Wen PY. Neurologic emergencies in cancer patients. *Neurol Clin* 1998;16:449–483.
41. Sørensen S, Børgesen SE, Rohde K, et al. Metastatic epidural spinal cord compression: results of treatment and survival. *Cancer* 1990;65:1502–1508.
42. Sørensen S, Helweg-Larsen S, Mouridsen H, Hansen HH. Effect of high-dose dexamethasone in carcinomatous metastatic spinal cord compression treated with radiotherapy: a randomized trial. *Eur J Cancer* 1994;30A:22–27.
43. Tancioni F, Navarria P, Lorenzetti MA, et al. Multimodal approach to the management of metastatic epidural spinal cord compression (MESCC) due to solid tumors. *Int J Radiat Oncol Biol Phys* 2010;78:1467–1473.
44. Vecht CJ, Haaxma-Reiche H, van Putten WL, et al. Initial bolus of conventional versus high-dose dexamethasone in metastatic spinal cord compression. *Neurology* 1989;39:1255–1257.
45. Wilson JR, Fehlings MG. Emerging approaches to the surgical management of acute traumatic spinal cord injury. *Neurotherapeutics* 2011;8:187–194.
46. Wong DA, Fornasier VL, MacNab I. Spinal metastases: the obvious, the occult, and the impostors. *Spine* 1990;15:1–4.
47. Yiu G, He Z. Glial inhibition of CNS axon regeneration. *Nat Rev Neurosci* 2006;7:617–627.

5

Treating Acute Autoimmune Encephalitis

Encephalitis is usually a result of a viral infection and has many mimickers. Recognizing that a clinical presentation might be consistent with acute encephalitis is just the first (and easy) step. Defining the precise cause of acute encephalitis is a much more difficult task that requires almost encyclopedic knowledge of neurologic and infectious disease. To put it simply, encephalitis can be infectious, postinfectious, and noninfectious. Equally important is to narrow the differential diagnosis depending on the season, geographic area, and specific exposures (including recent travel history) and other risk factors.

Neurologists—all over the world—have been confronted with a new, evolving disorder and are now handling a new difficult situation. Discovery of antineuronal antibodies led to further clinical characterization—what appears a mix of disorders,[23] Conditions that have been previously diagnosed as encephalitis of unknown cause are now categorized as paraneoplastic and autoimmune disorders.[2,17,20,22,39] but it is unclear whether there is an increase in incidence or an increase in recognition. Such a patient presents with an acute neurologic illness that rapidly evolves and requires a complex evaluation, aggressive treatment, and sometimes even exploratory surgery to find the culprit. The clinical presentation is highly worrisome, with a recognizable sequence of mild amnesia followed by confusion, a full encephalopathy syndrome followed by decreased level of consciousness, seizures, status epilepticus, and prolonged coma requiring intubation and mechanical ventilation. Cancers have been found, particularly ovarian teratomas, thymomas, or small-cell lung cancers, but many patients do not have identifiable tumors.

How do we approach a patient with an encephalitis? How do we recognize autoimmune encephalitis? How do we treat autoimmune encephalitis, how aggressively, and how long? This chapter describes this novel category of disorders associated with antibodies to neuronal cell surface antigens.[2,3,5–7,38] Many of these have only recently been discovered, and there are difficult decisions to be made. The recognition of autoimmune encephalitis pays off unconditionally, but here it is also placed in a wider category of encephalitis, providing a framework for an effective approach.

Principles

There are three core principles in assessing autoimmune encephalitis. One of the more interesting discoveries is that specific clinical features of autoimmune encephalitis have in some way or another been linked to specific antibodies (Table 5.1).[23] However, there is only tentative evidence that these antibody titers decline with improvement of the patient. Very few brain biopsies have been performed, with most abnormalities indistinctive. Biopsies are available in auto-immune encephalitides—and mostly the anti-N-methyl-D-aspartate receptor (NMDAR) variant—very few T-cell infiltrates are found, and only perivascular lymphocytic cuffing.

Several antibodies have now been characterized. These are antibodies against the entire receptor or components and are against NMDAR, gamma-aminobutyric acid type B (GABA$_B$) receptors, CASPR2 antibodies, and antibodies against LGI1 and contactin-2 (Figure 5.1).[22] These antibodies are found in serum and in cerebrospinal fluid (CSF)—suggesting intrathecal production—and have been identified, using indirect immunohistochemistry, on rodent brain sections and binding on hippocampal neurons in culture. The antibodies against voltage-gated potassium channel complexes have been better characterized, and a more specific protein, LGI1, was found, mostly in the hippocampus and neocortex. CASPR2 protein is also a cell surface protein and a cell adhesion molecule that facilitates localization of the voltage-gated potassium channel complex at the neuronal juxtaparanodes. Contactin-2 is expressed in axons of glial cells throughout the CSF.

Once one knows the type of antibodies, the clinical syndromes are easier to pinpoint. Limbic encephalitis, associated with antibodies to LGI1 antibodies, has a clinical presentation of worsening memory loss, confusion, seizures, agitation, and a variety of psychiatric signs and symptoms. It is more common in men older than 40 years. In this disorder, agitation is intense and difficult to treat. In many patients—up to 60%—a severe hyponatremia has been noted. These patients also most often have abnormal signal intensities on MRI scans, particularly in the medial temporal lobes. However, overall the sensitivity of MRI scan is approximately 50%; and a PET scan may be able to find more hippocampal dysfunction.[11]

Movement disorders are more common in patients with voltage-gated potassium channel antibodies (VGCK) and they may involve dystonia of face and arm.[27,33,37] Neuropsychiatric features always precede movement disorders, and autonomic dysfunction (often hypothermia) and abnormal consciousness follow about two weeks after onset. Limbic encephalitis associated with GABA$_B$ receptors and AMPA receptor antibodies does present with amnesia, as seen in limbic encephalitis, but with no clearly identifiable other clinical features.[15,18,20] Limbic

Table 5.1 **CNS antibody-associated disorders in adults**

	VGKC-Complex-Ab; Mainly LGI1-Abs	VGKC-Complex-Ab; Mainly CASPR2-Abs	Anti-NMDAR Encephalitis	AMPAR-Ab Limbic Encephalitis	GABA$_B$R-Ab Limbic Encephalitis	GAD-Ab Limbic Encephalitis	GlyR-Ab-Associated Disorders
Common symptoms	Limbic encephalitis with amnesia, seizures, psychiatric disturbance; faciobrachial dystonia	Morvan's phenotype with confusion, amnesia, insomnia, autonomic dysfunction, neuromyotonia	Multistage corticosubcortical encephalopathy including psychiatric manifestations, dyskinesias, seizures, mutism	Typical limbic encephalitis (amnesia, seizures); with prominent psychosis	Limbic encephalitis with prominent seizures	Temporal lobe epilepsy	Combinations of startle, rigidity, brainstem findings
Tumor association or other pathology	Tumors very rare	Thymoma or small cell lung cancer	Ovarian (or other) teratomas	Thymoma, lung, breast	Thymoma, lung	Very uncommon	Usually nonparaneoplastic
Disease course	Often monophasic without need for continuing immunosuppression	Treatment-responsive or spontaneous improvement	Responds to early immunotherapies and early tumor removal	Responds to treatments but relapses common	Responds to treatments	Usually chronic disorders	Immunotherapy with substantial improvement

VGKC = voltage-gated potassium channel. Ab = antibody. LGI1 = leucine-rich glioma inactivated 1. NMDAR = NMDA receptor. AMPAR = AMPA receptor. GABA$_B$R = GABA type B receptor. GAD = glutamic acid decarboxylase. GlyR = glycine receptor. CASPR2 = contactin associated protein 2.

Source: Adapted from references 6–8, 37

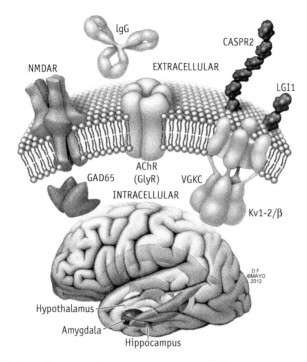

Figure 5.1 Main antigens causing autoimmune encephalitis.

encephalitis associated with glutamic acid decarboxylase (GAD) antibodies may present with stiff-man syndrome, cerebellar ataxia, or recurrent seizures.

Anti-NMDAR encephalitis is the encephalitis that has been most recently investigated. These antibodies are directed to one subunit of the NMDAR and are mostly found in CSF. Many patients have intrathecal synthesis of these antibodies, and the diagnosis therefore may be inaccurately discarded as a possibility if serum titers are negative and CSF is not investigated for antibodies. Anti-NMDAR encephalitis affects young women with ovarian teratomas. Finding these teratomas, which may have neuronal cells that could incite the neuroimmunologic response, may require aggressive screening and, in some instances with refractory clinical manifestations, ovariectomy. Removal of the tumor has been linked to rapid improvement and much better prognosis. CT scan of the abdomen and pelvis, as well as ultrasound, may reveal normal-appearing ovaries, but after salpingo-oophorectomy one may find small nests of teratoma cells.

A second core principle is that these disorders respond to immunomodulating treatments. Many of these patients progress to status epilepticus that is difficult to treat and the main reason for admission to a neurologic intensive care unit. It is logical to assume that status epilepticus can be controlled only after the encephalitis is controlled with aggressive chemotherapy. The fact that plasma exchange improves the condition argues that these antibodies are pathognomonic, and better results have sometimes been found with rituximab or cyclophosphamide, which can actually breach the blood-brain barrier.

Many other antibodies have been found with limbic encephalitis. Most of them are characterized as HU, MA2, and CRMP-5. Patients with anti-HU antibodies mostly have a small cell lung carcinoma and may present with refractory complex partial status epilepticus. Patients with anti-CRMP-5 antibodies present mostly with myelitis, optic neuritis, cerebellar ataxia, and uveitis. The disorder seems to be extending beyond the limbic system and involves the basal ganglia. Anti-MA2 encephalitis is often seen in males with germ cell tumors of the testes.[9] Similar to anti-NMDAR encephalitis, this would require aggressive evaluation and may require testicular removal to demonstrate microscopic tumors.

Another rare syndrome that has been associated with antibodies against the voltage-gated potassium channel is Morvan syndrome. These patients mostly have prominent dysautonomia, REM sleep disturbances, and hyponatremia.[19,24,30] Many patients develop significant hypothermia, hypersalivation, and a variety of psychiatric symptoms that include hallucinations. A small minority of patients will have underlying tumors, and then lung cancer is usually found.

In Practice

Autoimmune encephalitis is rare, and therefore other causes of viral encephalitis have to be carefully investigated. Even if the clinical features are characteristic, it might be difficult to see the forest for the trees and where to start and what to test.[1,12–15,31] A recent study of acute encephalitis notably found that most encephalitides in Asia were due to Japanese encephalitis; in Africa, due to rabies; and in Europe, due to varicella-zoster virus in children and due to tick-borne encephalitis virus in adults. A large number of encephalitis is uncharacterized.[13]

WORKING UP ENCEPHALITIS

In many countries, viral infection is the most common cause of acute encephalitis in adults. Epidemic outbreaks are produced by the seasonal spread of arboviruses (i.e., viruses transmitted by arthropod vectors, such as mosquitoes).[31] Most of these encephalitides are constrained to specific geographical locations; but there are exceptions such as the West Nile virus, which has been identified as a cause of summer outbreaks of encephalitis on all continents.[29]

Herpes simplex virus 1 (HSV-1) is a cause of sporadic viral encephalitis in immunocompetent patients. Albeit rare when all causes are taken into account, herpes simplex encephalitis remains the most common and has no seasonality. Outcome is related to whether or not there has been treatment with intravenous acyclovir. HSV-1 encephalitis has a predilection for the temporal lobes, insula, and operculum. Consequently, it should be suspected when febrile patients develop confusion or drowsiness associated with seizures or focal deficits referable to those locations. When present, the typical distribution of swelling on brain MRI strongly supports the diagnosis. However, the diagnosis should be established by confirming the presence of the virus in the CSF. Polymerase chain reaction (PCR) can detect HSV-1 DNA in the CSF with great sensitivity and specificity. If PCR is negative but the clinical-radiological presentation is suspicious for HSV-1 infection, the test should be repeated on a new CSF sample.

Other herpes viruses are even more uncommon in immunocompetent patients, but Epstein-Barr virus–associated encephalitis is regularly described in children. Varicella-zoster virus (VZV) occurs in approximately 2 out of 100,000 cases, usually presenting as ataxia emerging into a more diffuse encephalitis. VZV encephalitis in adults is often reactivation after use of corticosteroids. It may present as a vasculopathy or as a lymphocytic meningoencephalitis. Cytomegalovirus is more common in developing countries and in immunodeficient patients, but the prevalence has declined thanks to treatment with antiretroviral therapy. All these herpes viruses can be detected by PCR. An important additional virus to consider is human herpesvirus 6 (HHV-6), which may clinically present as nearly identical to autoimmune encephalitis but is predominantly seen in transplant recipients. HHV-6 is the most common cause of post-transplant acute limbic encephalitis, usually among recipients of allogeneic stem cell transplantation.

Arboviruses are seasonal because they are transmitted by arthropods, mosquitoes, ticks, and flies. Best known are West Nile virus, tick-borne encephalitis and Japanese encephalitis typically presenting during summer outbreaks.[29,32] The disorder that might be comparable to autoimmune encephalitis (when considering worldwide exposure) is rabies caused by dog or bat bite. This is an extremely rare disorder, although the World Health Organization estimates about 55,000 yearly cases. Rabies encephalitis has prominent manifestations of dysautonomia (which makes it comparable to autoimmune encephalitis) and the classic hydrophobia (oropharyngeal spasm on attempting to drink water). In Western countries it is almost never diagnosed but often considered in unexplained cases. There are a number of other viral encephalitides associated with exposure to animals, predominantly rodents. Hanta virus encephalitis is usually preceded by a respiratory-renal syndrome and thrombocythemia, but the viral transmission is airborne. (In the United States, several cases were recently registered in Yosemite National Park.)

If the clinical presentation involves brainstem symptomatology, a rhombencephalitis due to listeria or JC virus should be considered. Progressive multifocal leukoencephalopathy (PML) is due to JC virus and may rapidly produce severe dysphagia, ophthalmoplegia, and spasticity. It has been linked to natalizumab-treated patients and the risk of developing PML is markedly increased in patients who have positive JC virus titers. There is no effective treatment other than reversing immunosuppression—which may be problematic too.[4]

Generally, any viral infection can lead to viral encephalitis or a postinfectious acute disseminated encephalomyelitis (ADEM). Clinically there are certain pointers for ADEM. These are constitutional symptoms 4 to 40 days before neurologic manifestations and often pyramidal signs, cranial nerve involvement, and spinal cord involvement. Differentiating acute viral encephalitis from ADEM can be very difficult on MRI—typically ADEM spares the U fibers, is not associated with leptomeningeal enhancement, and often evolves into fluffy, spotty lesions.

The evaluation of encephalitis can be very costly and may lead to nothing revealing. A guideline for possible tests—ordered when there is a high a priori probability—is shown in Table 5.2. Moreover, certain radiological features may point toward etiology (Table 5.3).

The treatment of many encephalitides is support only. In more severe cases of postinfectious origin, there is a rationale to use IV methyl prednisolone, IVIG, plasma exchange, or combinations.

TREATING ENCEPHALITIS

The management of acute encephalitis may require admission to an intensive care unit. Even when the cause of the encephalitis is not treatable, comprehensive supportive care increases the chance of a favorable outcome. The major issues are recognition and treatment of seizures requiring continuous video/EEG monitoring, intubation and mechanical ventilation in patients unable to protect the airway (due to marked dysautonomia-related secretions, abnormal consciousness, or requirement of anesthetic drugs). Patients could be admitted to treat a refractory agitation.

All patients with presumed acute encephalitis should be started immediately on intravenous acyclovir (10 mg/kg using ideal body weight every 8 hours and longer intervals between doses in patients with reduced glomerular filtration rate). This antiviral agent is the first choice for treating HSV-1, HSV-2, and VZV. Cytomegalovirus infection requires the combination of ganciclovir and foscarnet, but these patients should also be tested for HIV infection. HIV-infected patients must receive a highly active antiretroviral therapy. Ganciclovir and foscarnet are also the preferred treatment choices for HSV-6 infection in immunosuppressed patients. No antiviral has been proven effective against West Nile virus infection.

EEG is mandatory in patients with encephalitis. It is not infrequent to see seizures in patients who exhibit fluctuating levels of awareness, and 24-hour continuous EEG monitoring may provide useful information. Continuous EEG monitoring should also be considered in comatose patients with encephalitis. Nonconvulsive seizures are not uncommon but should be differentiated from interictal periodic lateralized epileptiform discharges (PLEDs). Nonconvulsive seizures must be treated with antiepileptic drugs. Only when PLEDS are frequent or tend to become rhythmic, antiepileptic drugs should be used to prevent seizures. However, adjusting the doses just to eliminate PLEDS has not been proven to work and often provokes drug toxicity, as these discharges tend to be quite refractory.

Brain biopsy in unexplained encephalitis is only considered when all noninvasive diagnostic alternatives have been tried. It is also advisable to search for other biopsy targets before invading the brain and there may be an easy location in the brain to

Table 5.2 **Tests Considered to Narrow Cause of Encephalitis**

Screen	Disease or agent tested
Infectious	*HSV I, *HSV II, *VZV, *EBV, *HHV6, *St. Louis Encephalitis virus, *Western Equine Encephalitis virus, *West Nile virus, *Eastern Equine Encephalitis, *Measles virus, *Enterovirus, *Adenovirus, *Influenza A, *Influenza B, *Chlamydia species, *Mycoplasma pneumoniae, *HIV, *RPR-VDRL, *Lyme serology, *CMV, JC virus, *Mycobacterium tuberculosis, Toxoplasma serology, Ehrlichia, Cryptococcus neoformans, *Bartonella, Fungal culture, prion disease, Rocky Mountain Spotted fever, Tularemia, Babesiosis, Hanta virus, Rabies.
Toxicological	Marijuana, *benzodiazepines, *amphetamines,*cocaine, LSD, heroin, PCP, ecstasy, heavy metals
Immunological	*ANA, *antithyroid antibodies, *anti-dsDNA, ANCA, Jo-1, Ro, La, Scl-70, Rheumatoid factor, *ESR, *C-reactive protein, serum ACE level, *CSF immunoelectrophoresis, *anti-GluR3, anti-GAD65, anti-VGKC antibody
Neoplastic	*CXR, *CT thorax, abdomen, pelvis, *whole body PET, bone marrow biopsy, *CSF cytology, *CSF flow cytometry
Paraneoplastic	*Anti-Hu, *Ma2, *CV2/CRMP5, *antiamphiphysin, *anti-VGKC, anti-NMDA receptor antibody
Metabolic	*Renal panel, *liver panel, *electrolytes, *Ca/Mg, *ammonia level, B12 level, folate, lactate, pyruvate, CPK, thyroid function, glucose, *porphyria screen, *celiac disease (anti-tTG, antiendomysium)
Hematologic	*CBC, blood smear, *hypercoagulable screen including anticardiolipin and antiphospholipid antibodies
Vascular	*CTA or MRA, *MR venography
Genetic	Skin and muscle biopsy, serum and CSF lactate and pyruvate, genetic screen for known MERRF and MELAS mutations, muscle respiratory chain enzyme assay, very long chain fatty acid screen, lysosomal enzyme screen, blood and urine amino acid screen, urine organic acid panel, serum copper and ceruloplasmin, urine sulfate, blood and urine urate levels, white cell enzyme studies, serum lipids, MR spectroscopy
Other	18-FDG PET brain, SPECT, Biopsy (meninges, cortex, white matter), saliva for rabies

*Tests highlighted by asterisk should be considered first. HIV: human immunodeficiency virus; RPR: rapid plasma reagin; VDRL: venereal disease research laboratory; HSV: herpes simplex virus; EBV: Epstein-Barr virus; CMV: cytomegalovirus; VZV: varicella-zoster virus; TB: tuberculosis; HHV: human herpesvirus; ANA: antinuclear antibody; dsDNA: double-stranded DNA; ANCA: anticytoplasmic antibody; GluR: glutamate receptor; GAD: glutamic acid decarboxylase; VGKC: voltage-gated potassium channel: CXR: chest X-ray; CT: computer tomography; PET: positron emission tomography; CSF: cerebrospinal fluid; NMDA: N-methyl-D-aspartic acid; CK: creatine kinase; MERRF: myoclonus epilepsy with ragged red fibers; MELAS: mitochondrial myopathy, encephalopathy, lactic acidosis, and stroke-like episodes; FDG: fluorodeoxyglucose; SPECT: single photon emission computed tomography.

Source: Reference 1, 13, 17.

Table 5.3 **Acute Encephalitis with Characteristic Radiological Features**

Cause	Characteristic Radiological Features
Herpes simplex virus type 1	Inflammatory lesions in temporal lobes, insula, and operculum
Varicella Zoster virus	Multifocal infarctions and irregularities of arterial lumen; nodular meningeal enhancement Cerebellitis in children
Epstein-Barr	Cortical, basal ganglia, and cerebellar hyperintensities on MRI
Cytomegalovirus	Ventriculitis (subependymal enhancement). Brainstem inflammation
West Nile virus	Myelitis*
Tuberculosis	Basilar meningitis[†]
Fungal infections	Abscess formation**
Autoimmune limbic encephalitis	Inflammatory lesions in mesial temporal lobes
Acute disseminated encephalomyelitis	Bilateral white matter T2-hyperintense lesions. Corpus callosum involvement
Progressive multifocal leucoencephalopathy (JC virus)	Bilateral, confluent T2-hyperintense lesions in temporo-occipital white matter with involvement of U fibers and cortical sparing

*Presentation with acute flaccid paralysis may occur with or without radiological signs of myelitis.
[†]Also with fungal meningoencephalitis caused by *Blastomycosis*
**Aspergillus* species is characterized by cerebral infarctions and hemorrhages

go after. Detailed physical examination with special attention to the skin and lymph node chains; CT scans of chest, abdomen, and pelvis; and PET scan can reveal a more accessible site for tissue sampling. The evaluation and treatment of autoimmune encephalitis is different from that of other encephalitides. The responsibility is an immediate, aggressive workup that include evaluation with MRI of the brain and EEG monitoring.[10] In younger patients teratoma are more common, in older patients carcinoma are more common although only found in some patients.[36] CT of the abdomen and pelvis, a PET scan, and biopsy in uncertain lesions is needed.

Treatment in autoimmune encephalitis is often initially 5 to 10 infusions of IV immunoglobulin, 5 to 10 sessions of plasma exchange,[26] and 1 gram of methylprednisolone for 5 to 10 days. In many patients, seizures can only be controlled when the disease is treated more aggressively using a combination of rituximab and cyclophosphamide.[8,25] Rituximab is usually used in a dose of 375 mg/m^2 every week for 4 weeks and combined with cyclophosphamide 750 mg/m^2 given with the first dose of rituximab, which is then followed by monthly cycles of cyclophosphamide.[6] Oral cyclophosphamide or intravenous cyclophosphamide will lead to hair loss and bone marrow suppression (marked neutropenia days after administration, as expected in most chemotherapeutic agents). Both rituximab and cyclophosphamide are effective many weeks after administration and, thus, an early effect cannot be expected. Aggressive and prolonged treatment of status epilepticus might be necessary, and there have been full recoveries in patients who have been treated for several months.[16,17,35] However, outcome in others are less favorable, with refractory status epilepticus in several patients despite ovariectomy and combinations of rituximab and cyclophosphamide. Many expert feel it is important to continue aggressive and sustained immunotherapy for several months to allow improvement.

By the Way

- Autoimmune encephalitis is usually diagnosed by CSF antibody titers
- Outcome in autoimmune encephalitis depends on control of status epilepticus
- Outcome in autoimmune encephalitis in patients older than 50 years may be much worse
- Outcome in autoimmune encephalitis improves after removal of a teratoma, seminoma, or single small cell cancer mass

---

Encephalitis By the Numbers

- ~90% of autoimmune encephalitis have potential for good outcome
- ~80% of the time no causative agent is found in encephalitis
- ~70% of patients with encephalitis have seizures or status epilepticus
- ~70% of patients with arboviral encephalitis have a poor outcome
- ~50% of patients with HSV encephalitis have good outcome
- ~10% of encephalitis is due to herpes simplex virus
- ~10% of encephalitis is fungal

Putting It All Together

- Arboviral encephalitis is most prevalent cause of encephalitis, and West Nile virus is the arbovirus most commonly encountered in the United States
- Paraneoplastic and autoimmune encephalitis are newly emerging disorders
- MRI often yields negative results in encephalitis

- Intravenous acyclovir is an appropriate empiric treatment until the HSV-PCR result becomes available
- Aggressive care of autoimmune encephalitis may lead to good outcome despite initially worrisome neurologic findings

References

1. Ambrose HE, Granerod J, Clewley JP, et al. Diagnostic strategy used to establish etiologies of encephalitis in a prospective cohort of patients in England. *J Clin Microbiol* 2011;49:3576–3583.
2. Armangue T, Petit-Pedrol M, Dalmau J. Autoimmune encephalitis in children. *J Child Neurol* 2012;27:1460–1469.
3. Buckley C, Vincent A. Autoimmune channelopathies. *Nat Clin Pract Neurol* 2005;1:22–33.
4. Chen Y, Bord E, Tompkins T, et al. Asymptomatic reactivation of JC virus in patients treated with natalizumab. *N Engl J Med* 2009;361:1067–1074.
5. Costello DJ, Kilbride RD, Cole AJ. Cryptogenic new onset refractory status epilepticus (NORSE) in adults—infectious or not? *J Neurol Sci* 2009;277:26–31.
6. Dalmau J, Gleichman AJ, Hughes EG, et al. Anti-NMDA-receptor encephalitis: case series and analysis of the effects of antibodies. *Lancet Neurol* 2008;7:1091–1098.
7. Dalmau J, Lancaster E, Martinez-Hernandez E, Rosenfeld MR, Balice-Gordon R. Clinical experience and laboratory investigations in patients with anti-NMDAR encephalitis. *Lancet Neurol* 2011;10:63–74.
8. Dalmau J, Rosenfeld MR. Paraneoplastic syndromes of the CNS. *Lancet Neurol* 2008;7:327–340.
9. Dalmau J. Status epilepticus due to paraneoplastic and nonparaneoplastic encephalitides. *Epilepsia* 2009;50:58–60.
10. Day GS, High SM, Cot B, Tang-Wai DF. Anti-NMDA-receptor encephalitis: case report and literature review of an under-recognized condition. *J Gen Intern Med* 2011;26:811–816.
11. Demaerel P, Van Dessel W, Van Paesschen W, et al. Autoimmune-mediated encephalitis. *Neuroradiology* 2011;53:837–851.
12. Gilden D, Cohrs RJ, Mahalingam R, Nagel MA. Varicella zoster virus vasculopathies: diverse clinical manifestations, laboratory features, pathogenesis, and treatment. *Lancet Neurol* 2009;8:731–740.
13. Glaser CA, Honarmand S, Anderson LJ, et al. Beyond viruses: clinical profiles and etiologies associated with encephalitis. *Clin Infect Dis* 2006;43:1565–1577.
14. Granerod J, Cunningham R, Zuckerman M, et al. Causality in acute encephalitis: defining etiologies. *Epidemiol Infect* 2010;138:783–800.
15. Granerod J, Tam CC, Crowcroft NS, et al. Challenge of the unknown: a systematic review of acute encephalitis in non-outbreak situations. *Neurology* 2010;75:924–932.
16. Graus F, Boronat A, Xifro X, et al. The expanding clinical profile of anti-AMPA receptor encephalitis. *Neurology* 2010;74:857–859.
17. Iizuka T, Sakai F, Ide T, et al. Anti-NMDA receptor encephalitis in Japan: long-term outcome without tumor removal. *Neurology* 2008;70:504–511.
18. Iizuka T, Sakai F, Mochizuki H. Update on anti-NMDA receptor encephalitis. *Brain Nerve* 2010;62:331–338.
19. Irani SR, Alexander S, Waters P, et al. Antibodies to Kv1 potassium channel-complex proteins leucine-rich, glioma inactivated 1 protein and contactin-associated protein-2 in limbic encephalitis, Morvan's syndrome and acquired neuromyotonia. *Brain* 2010;133:2734–2748.
20. Jacob S, Irani SR, Rajabally YA, et al. Hypothermia in VGKC antibody-associated limbic encephalitis. *J Neurol Neurosurg Psychiatry* 2008;79:202–204.

21. Jubelt B, Mihai C, Li TM, Veerapaneni P. Rhombencephalitis/brainstem encephalitis. *Curr Neurol Neurosci Rep*. 2011;11:543–552.
22. Lai M, Huijbers MG, Lancaster E, et al. Investigation of LGI1 as the antigen in limbic encephalitis previously attributed to potassium channels: a case series. *Lancet Neurol* 2010;9:776–785.
23. Lancaster E, Martinez-Hernandez E, Dalmau J. Encephalitis and antibodies to synaptic and neuronal cell surface proteins. *Neurology* 2011;77:179–189.
24. Liguori R, Vincent A, Clover L, et al. Morvan's syndrome: peripheral and central nervous system and cardiac involvement with antibodies to voltage-gated potassium channels. *Brain* 2001;124:2417–2426.
25. Petereit HF, Rubbert-Roth A. Rituximab levels in cerebrospinal fluid of patients with neurological autoimmune disorders. *Mult Scler* 2009;15:189–192.
26. Pham HP, Daniel-Johnson JA, Stotler BA, Stephens H, Schwartz J. Therapeutic plasma exchange for the treatment of anti-NMDA receptor encephalitis. *J Clin Apher* 2011;26:320–325.
27. Pozo-Rosich P, Clover L, Saiz A, Vincent A, Graus F. Voltage-gated potassium channel antibodies in limbic encephalitis. *Ann Neurol* 2003;54:530–533.
28. Prüss H, Dalmau J, Harms L, et al. Retrospective analysis of NMDA receptor antibodies in encephalitis of unknown origin. *Neurology* 2010;75:1735–1739.
29. Rossi SL, Ross TM, Evans JD. West Nile virus. *Clin Lab Med* 2010;30:47–65.
30. Serratrice G, Serratrice J. Continuous muscle activity, Morvan's syndrome and limbic encephalitis: ionic or non ionic disorders? *Acta Myol* 2011;30:32–33.
31. Stahl JP, Mailles A, Dacheux L, Morand P. Epidemiology of viral encephalitis in 2011. *Med Mal Infect* 2011;41:453–464.
32. Süss J. Tick-borne encephalitis 2010: epidemiology, risk areas, and virus strains in Europe and Asia-an overview. *Ticks Tick Borne Dis* 2011;2:2–15.
33. Tan KM, Lennon VA, Klein CJ, Boeve BF, Pittock SJ. Clinical spectrum of voltage-gated potassium channel autoimmunity. *Neurology* 2008;70:1883–1890.
34. Thieben MJ, Lennon VA, Boeve BF, Aksamit AJ, Keegan M, Vernino S. Potentially reversible autoimmune limbic encephalitis with neuronal potassium channel antibody. *Neurology* 2004;62:1177–1182.
35. Titulaer MJ, McCracken L, Gabilondo I, et al. Treatment and prognostic factors for long-term outcome in patients with anti-NMDA receptor encephalitis: an observational cohort study *Lancet* 2013;12:157–165.
36. Titulaer MJ, McCracken L, Gabilondo I, et al. Late-onset anti-NMDA receptor encephalitis *Neurology* 2013;17:1058–1063.
37. Vincent A, Buckley C, Schott JM, et al. Potassium channel antibody-associated encephalopathy: a potentially immunotherapy-responsive form of limbic encephalitis. *Brain* 2004;127:701–712.
38. Vincent A, Lang B, Kleopa KA. Autoimmune channelopathies and related neurological disorders. *Neuron* 2006;52:123–138.
39. Wingfield T, McHugh C, Vas A, Richardson A, et al. Autoimmune encephalitis: a case series and comprehensive review of the literature. *QJM* 2011;104:921–931.

6

Neurosurgical Emergencies in Acute Brain Injury

Acute brain injury may be stable or deteriorating and at any point could require attention by a neurosurgeon. As expected, the more severely injured patients are immediately triaged to neurosurgical or surgical trauma services. When such a patient arrives in the emergency room, often a neurologist and a neurosurgeon will automatically see the patient, but not necessarily together. In tertiary centers, the emergency physician, neurointensivist, or neurologist will assess the patient on arrival. Naturally, a neurologist must recognize tip-over situations and know when it is necessary to involve a neurosurgeon.

A wide range of conditions must—without hesitation—result in an emergency page to the neurosurgeon on call. In traumatic brain injury (TBI), this applies in most instances to situations where there are CT-visible contusions or subdural or epidural hematoma, but it also applies to cerebral hemorrhage with mass effect, aneurysmal subarachnoid hemorrhage, any swollen stroke, acute subdural empyema, or shunt malfunction. More specifically, a cerebral hematoma—due to a ruptured intracranial aneurysm, arteriovenous malformation, or fistula—introduces an additional set of problems and dilemmas. Once emergency neurosurgery is started and a vascular malformation is discovered, neurosurgeons may be facing a bigger problem.

Immediate highly effective interventions include placement of a ventriculostomy for acute hydrocephalus in an obstructing tumor, intraventricular hemorrhage, or subarachnoid hemorrhage. In many patients with a poor grade subarachnoid hemorrhage acute hydrocephalus is a contributing factor, and intraventricular hemorrhage is often present. Placement of a ventriculostomy, particularly at drainage levels between 5 and 10 mm Hg, will maintain an open drain and reduce intracranial pressure. Long-term aggressive drainage can be performed after the aneurysm has been secured through coiling or clipping.

There are several ways of approaching these patients, and there are differences of approach among neurosurgeons. As in any surgical procedure, there might be neurosurgeons that are quick to respond and others who are more conservative—what matters is what makes the most sense. Neurosurgical preferences may be guided by the presence of a lesion in the non-dominant hemisphere, good rehabilitation potential before surgery, and most certainly absence of a moribund condition or end-stage illness such as advanced cancer, kidney or liver disease. Many neurosurgeons feel that evacuation of any acute lesion causing mass effect is warranted—others would want to wait until the patient deteriorates, knowingly accepting the risk that the patient might have too much secondary injury to benefit from surgery. An underappreciated factor is that patients may have deteriorated during transport and this may not be clear at first sight. Even in hospitals in close proximity, the delay during the daytime may still be substantial, which may allow patients to deteriorate when there is no opportunity for specialty care. This is a result of finding a tertiary center with an available bed, obtaining consent of the patient or family, and arranging for adequate transport.[2,3]

Why is acute neurosurgical intervention effective in evacuation of a new brain mass and why is it not in some cases? What are the emergency neurosurgical procedures in acute brain injury that physicians should be familiar with? How crucial is timing of surgery? This chapter reviews these neurosurgical options.

Principles

A good understanding of principles is needed to explain potential outcomes following an emergency evacuation of a new lesion. There are several factors, all having to do with fairly simple mechanics. Neurosurgical evacuation of a lesion creates space and results in less compression of the diencephalon (thalamus), or less shift or buckling of the upper brainstem. Less mass effect may also result in less risk for ischemic injury due to displacement of brainstem vasculature.[29] There may also be regional effects surrounding the mass that could determine outcome.

The question why neurosurgical evacuation could possibly improve outcome in intracerebral hemorrhage can also be deduced from understanding the mechanism of brain injury in this condition. There are multiple mechanisms to consider. First, the presence of mass effect initially may cause the middle of the brain to be squeezed underneath the falx, compressing the anterior cerebral artery. Second—the most important effect—is further translation of force toward the upper brainstem. Shift of the brainstem will cause tethering of the arteries and abnormal perfusion of the brainstem and may tear smaller penetrating arteries, which may cause secondary hemorrhages, make the injury permanent, and worsen the probability of recovery. These injuries are much less obvious than the so-called Duret hemorrhage and do not show on regular CT scans. Duret hemorrhages are most typically induced by a sudden, rapid, dramatic increase in cerebrospinal fluid (CSF) pressure injuring the periventricular lining.

What is unclear and unresolved is what happens in tissue surrounding the mass (or clot) under pressure. Is that tissue ischemic, temporarily non-functional, or even apoptotic? A commonly held notion is that compression effects cause a perihematomal ischemic penumbra, but such an explanation was not supported by experimental studies.[24] If the cerebral metabolic rate of oxygen and oxygen extraction fraction is examined using PET scanning, these parameters were reduced in the perihematomal region, suggesting a zone of hypoperfusion but without ischemia.[29] Studies have shown that the perihematoma region is basically a zone of low cerebral blood flow left after early clot retraction.[31,37]

What other effects does a clot have on surrounding brain tissue? One "toxic" substance might be thrombin that frees itself as a result of clot formation.[5,9] Thrombin may induce apoptosis and potentiate glutamate. Thrombin-induced brain edema is the result of opening of the blood-brain barrier.[10,11,19,35] When thrombin is removed in experimental studies, perihematomal edema does not occur. Drugs such as argatroban, a thrombin inhibitor, appear to reduce cerebral edema following intracranial hemorrhage in animal experiments.[8,13,15] (It seems that as an anticoagulant, argatroban is a double-edged sword.)

Another focus of interest by research groups is the potential toxic effect of iron in hemoglobin that will increase reactive oxygen species and cause additional brain damage.[36] Any new lesion could also incite an inflammatory response and increase matrix metalloproteinase. These enzymes can disrupt the blood-brain barrier and cause cerebral edema. One can, therefore, imagine that future therapies should concentrate on reducing the clot size, which could reduce the inflammatory and toxic effect of thrombin and iron, or minimize the effect of blood by draining it through a ventriculostomy.[36]

Timing of surgery may be relevant, because parenchymal hematomas expand from rebleeding, and they do most of their expansion within 6 hours after the initial arterial bleeding has stopped. In approximately a third of patients, hematomas expand and it appears that a reasonable estimate can be made of how much hematoma expansion will occur.[1,28] A simple approach is to divide the total volume by the time in hours. This time is onset of symptoms to CT scanning. A hematoma growth ratio of more than 10 does increase the probability of further enlargement.[28]

What is the role of blood pressure control? Current trials are testing the effect of early aggressive blood pressure control and may provide answers, but the "blood pressure/hematoma enlargement" issue has remained unresolved. Aggressive and early control of blood pressure has recently been associated with development of abnormal lesions, depicted by diffusion-weighted imaging (DWI), surrounding and remote from the hemorrhage site.[6,22] Although experimental studies have not been able to document a penumbra in intracerebral hematomas, aggressive blood pressure reduction could lead to ischemic injury in marginally perfused areas.

Mass effect may occur from recent cerebral infarction. Two conditions potentially warrant acute neurosurgical advice. Acute infarcts in the cerebellum may compress the brainstem and then often compress the fourth ventricle, resulting in obstructive hydrocephalus. These two mechanisms go together and require two interventions—suboccipital decompression and a ventriculostomy. Decompressive craniotomy is also warranted in any massive hemispheric infarction with early edema, and "creating space" is the only option to reduce mass effect. The evolution of mass effect is unpredictable—often protracted, sometimes rapid—and no neurosurgeon wants to guess here.

The same options pertain to situations where a lesion cannot be removed, such as in diffuse axonal injury. Decompressive craniectomy allows swelling of the brain outside the skull. It is a misunderstanding that this type of surgery would always be beneficial, because swelling is in all directions and can still be damaging. Decompressive craniectomy can reduce intracranial pressure, but release of pressure may also initially aggravate the development of brain edema. Acute decompression increases transcapillary hydrostatic pressure and could potentially promote development of vasogenic edema.

In Practice

The relationship of neurologists, neurointensivists, or emergency physicians with a neurosurgeon works in a patient's favor. Each provides something the other has to offer. So where does that leave the patient? There are few important and common clinical scenarios to discuss.

Mass effect may be associated with acute parenchymal hematoma. The neurosurgical decision to evacuate a hematoma is typically determined by worsening clinical signs.[23,25,27] The general consensus among neurosurgeons is that surgical evacuation of the deep-seated intracranial hematoma *does not* improve outcome, surgical evacuation for lobar hematoma located close to the surface *could* improve outcome, and surgical evacuation of a cerebellar hematoma *will* improve outcome. Neurosurgical intervention requires the documented presence of normal coagulation parameters, and patients may need additional treatment that could potentially delay the procedure. Patients with no evidence of comorbidities, an absence of ongoing anticoagulation or need for anticoagulation, and no evidence of intraventricular hemorrhage or secondary brainstem injury are ideal candidates.[26] Outcome after cerebral amyloid angiopathy-associated hemorrhage is not different from other types of hemorrhages, and there is no increased risk of re-exploration as a result of rehemorrhage.[20]

In any lobar hematoma, a cerebral angiogram or CT angiogram (CTA) is necessary to exclude an intracranial aneurysm or arteriovenous malformation (AVM) before proceeding further. Clot evacuation of the temporal lobe hematoma may be more often associated with a middle cerebral (bifurcation) aneurysm, but most CT scans will usually show additional hemorrhage in the basal cisterns, pointing toward an aneurysmal cause of the hematoma. Small AVMs or cavernous hemangiomas can be hidden inside the hematoma and may not be imaged by CTA.

Another option is to place a ventriculostomy in a patient with cerebral hematoma and enlarged ventricles. The clinical setting in which ventriculostomy is most often considered is in a patient with a thalamic hematoma or caudate hemorrhage that easily ruptures into the ventricular system. Larger clots with interventricular hemorrhage obviously are associated with coma and loss of upper brainstem reflexes, and often extension of the hematoma not only into the ventricles but also into the diencephalon, increasing the chance of a permanent injury and poor outcome. Ventriculostomy would allow for aggressive drainage of interventricular hemorrhage and the possibility of injection of thrombolytics. The fact is that most ventriculostomies placed in patients with hemorrhage into the ventricles will clot off quickly without the use of thrombolytics. Thrombolytics alone improve CT scan images with intraventricular hemorrhage, but whether improved outcome is due to the ability to continuously drain CSF and reduce intracranial pressure, or whether thrombolytics reduce intracranial hemorrhage and the secondary effects of hemorrhage is not fully resolved.

Emergency evacuation in patients with a lobar hematoma who have already lost upper brainstem reflexes is an area of contention. Patients presenting with lobar hematomas and loss of pupil and corneal reflexes rarely do well. This presentation may be a result of failure to recognize earlier signs of deterioration. One can thus make the argument that any patient who has deteriorated from a lobar hematoma—even if the clinical difference is subtle—should have a neurosurgical intervention. Clinical deterioration in lobar hematoma is more common than appreciated; for example, in the famed STICH trial, 1 in 4 patients who were initially treated medically deteriorated, requiring surgical evacuation.[17] The STICH-II results—again in non-deteriorating patients with superficial lobar hemorrhages—showed no benefit except in a subset with no intraventricular hemorrhage.[18] It remains unclear if these results will change practice and most neurosurgeons have a low threshold to take out easily accessible hematomas with any hint of worsening.

When an aneurysm is found in a patient with a large expansile temporal lobe hematoma, several options are possible. The hematoma is usually initially removed and, if feasible, clipped at the same time. Many middle cerebral artery aneurysms are at the bifurcation, with a wide base, incorporating important tributaries, and therefore cannot be considered for endovascular coil embolization. If the CTA shows a possible aneurysm that could be treated with coil embolization, this procedure should follow immediately after the hematoma evacuation. Endovascular coiling of an aneurysm while a hematoma is present may be associated with deterioration during coil embolization.

Cerebellar hematomas are a neurosurgical emergency, although rarely "observation" can be considered. A "tight posterior fossa sign" on CT scan justifies early evacuation. This CT scan feature is defined as absent prepontine cisterns, inability to identify the fourth ventricle, acute hydrocephalus, or obliteration of the supracerebellar cisterns—these are all indications for clot evacuation. The fourth ventricle will recoil almost immediately after decompression, and the patient may improve in a matter of days. Bradycardia or episodic hypertension, not necessarily at the same time, indicate medulla oblongata compression from tonsillar coning or lateral displacement. Patients exhibiting these signs are at particular risk of further deterioration. Generally, one should appreciate that patients with a cerebellar hematoma can rapidly deteriorate and may lose all brainstem function in a matter of hours or minutes—evacuation may not result in a functional improvement. Thus, surgery is mandatory and "observation" can only be considered in the absence of mass effect (mostly when there is considerable cerebellar atrophy).

Mass effect may be associated with acute traumatic contusions or extraparenchymal hematomas. Neurosurgical treatment may involve evacuation of acute epidural or acute subdural hematoma, evacuation of a contusional lesion, perhaps also repair of depressed skull fractures or decompressive craniectomy, and, not infrequently, a combination of these surgical interventions. Several prospective trials have found that early versus late craniectomy after traumatic brain injury may not make a significant difference in outcome.[34] It is more important how care is provided after the surgical intervention and this includes careful fluid management, infection surveillance and antibiotic coverage if needed, surveillance for deep venous thrombosis, and early tracheostomy and gastrostomy to improve patients' recovery potential.

The decision to evacuate a contusion is determined by its size and mass effect. Current guidelines of the Congress of Neurological Surgeons and Brain Trauma Foundation include patients in coma (defined as Glasgow coma sum scores of 6–8) and a temporal or frontal contusion of larger than 20 cc with a midline shift of at least 5 mm or cisternal compression on CT. Patients with a lesion of 50 cc or greater would need surgery no matter what. It is further advised that only asymptomatic patients or patients "with little neurologic signs" and no mass effect on CT could be closely monitored with serial CT scans. Acute subdural hematoma of more than 10 mm or a midline shift of more than 5 mm should be removed surgically. A subdural hematoma becomes subacute in 2 weeks, and evacuation is determined by neurologic deficits that may include changes in cognition or severe persistent headache. Epidural hematomas are immediately treated surgically, and very few allow close observation—and then it is not clear which patient would qualify for a watchful approach. This may be in patients with less than 5-mm midline shift with no major neurologic deficit or change in level of consciousness.

How these recommendations to treat traumatic lesions translate to practice is not known and still leaves open a nonoperative approach to some patients, with intervention only if mass effect or volume of the contusion increases. Most neurosurgeons would have a low threshold if there were an accompanying subdural hematoma and would proceed with evacuation and, not infrequently, with decompressive craniectomy if further cerebral edema were anticipated.

UNILATERAL CRANIECTOMY   BILATERAL CRANIECTOMY

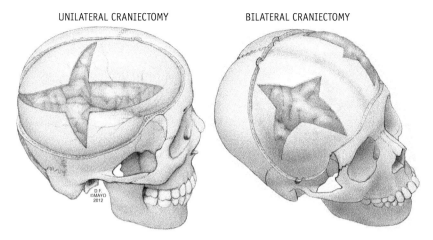

Figure 6.1 Unilateral and bilateral decompressive craniectomy. The cruciate incision for decompression is followed by oversewing with a collagen-based dural substitute and gelatin film barrier.

Under all these circumstances, neurosurgeons will proceed by placing the burr hole at the temporal end of the horseshoe-shaped incision and extending rapidly to allow decompression of a subdural hematoma or mass effect.

Decompressive craniectomy is a large bone flap and ideally should include decompression of the floor of the temporal fossa. The procedure of decompressive craniectomy for a traumatic head injury remains an arbitrary one and typically involves bifrontal decompression (Figures 6.1 and 6.2). Decompressive craniectomy is reserved for the more severely affected patients, because later cranioplasty is also associated with significant complications that include breakthrough seizures, subgaleal collections, wound infections, hydrocephalus, and osteomyelitis.[30,33]

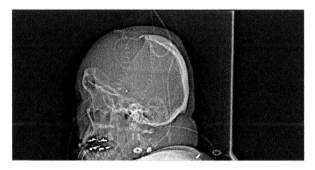

Figure 6.2 Bilateral decompressive craniectomy.

Decompressive craniectomy to treat refractory increased intracranial pressure for diffuse traumatic brain injury has been studied in detail.[7,21,32,33] The DECRA study found that early bifronto-temporoparietal decompressive craniectomy decreased intracranial pressure and length of stay but increased unfavorable outcome.[4] The study has been criticized, and questions were raised about the operative technique, the long accrual time suggesting that major differences in treatment might have occurred, and the fact that more patients with bilateral unreactive pupils were in the surgical group. The most concerning observation of this trial was that only minimal elevations to intracranial pressure prompted surgical management, mostly at the upper limit of normal at 20 mm Hg. (Most neurosurgeons would intervene with ICP spikes or progressive increase in ICP.)

The options are limited in the case of gunshot wounds. Destruction of the diencephalon, a track involving both hemispheres, early emerging cerebral edema, or a laceration of a major cerebral vessel leading to massive cerebral hematoma all implicitly point to a poor outcome or low likelihood of improvement. Removal of bone and bullet fragments in patients who are still responding (simply defined as localizing to pain and eye opening to pain) may be warranted in certain circumstances but not in those with lost pupil and corneal reflexes. Removal of bullet material lodged deep inside the brain or ventricles is rarely successful. However, the presence of pneumocephalus, epidural, or subdural hematomas, or subarachnoid hemorrhage should not sway a neurosurgeon to hold back.

There are several other conditions that warrant urgent neurosurgical evaluation and should be briefly discussed here. Any new or acute hydrocephalus—de novo observation or shunt malfunction—requires an urgent assessment. Some patients with acute hydrocephalus have a compressive tumor that needs further differentiation with MRI and later treatment. Ventriculoperitoneal shunt failure may present with stupor preceded by headache and emesis. Any episode of fever (and certainly recurrent temperature spikes) should prompt blood and CSF cultures and immediate broad-spectrum antibiotics before shunt revision. Shunt malfunction may be due to blockage of the ventricular catheter drainage openings, kinking or breakage of the abdominally placed catheter (in particular in patients with epilepsy), or, more fundamentally, underdrainage or overdrainage. Overdrainage may lead to progressive subdural effusion or hematomas; underdrainage will show progressive hydrocephalus with periventricular effusions or CT scans. Shunt malfunctions require revision but only after connections have been established with plain X-rays showing the tubing is intact (more details are in volume *Recognizing Brain Injury*).

The most troublesome, but fortunately rare, neurosurgical emergency is pituitary apoplexy, which usually presents with severe unrelenting headache and visual loss. Pituitary apoplexia occurs in pituitary adenoma, a tumor abundantly

Table 6.1 **When to Contact a Neurosurgeon in Acute Situations**

Condition	Procedure
• Subarachnoid hemorrhage	Aneurysmal repair (clip, coil, pipeline)
	Ventriculostomy for acute hydrocephalus
• Cerebral hematoma	Evacuation
	Ventriculostomy
• Hemispheric ischemic swelling	Decompressive craniectomy
• Traumatic brain injury	Craniotomy for contusion
	Craniectomy after penetrating injury
• Epidural empyema	Surgical evacuation and debridement
• Abscess	Drainage
• CSF leak	Repair of dural tear
• Shunt failure	Ventriculostomy
• Hemorrhage in pituitary tumor	Early surgical removal

supplied by hypophysial arteries and prone to bleed. Pituitary apoplexy may be the first presentation of the tumor, with clinical signs that range from trivial in nature to signs that are immediately life threatening. Most common is a headache that seems unexplained rapidly followed by visual field deficits or emerging third and sixth nerve palsies. Sudden proptosis is a very suspicious sign of compression of the cavernous sinus. CT scans may show a hyperdensity in the suprasellar region, but MRI is more diagnostic, albeit difficult to obtain quickly during presentation. Permanent visual deficits may occur if tumors compress the chiasm and when surgery is delayed.

To epitomize, acutely ill neurologic patients are never stable, and neurosurgical intervention should be anticipated. The most common reasons for emergency consultation with a neurosurgeon are summarized in Table 6.1.

By the Way

- International normalized ratio of less than 1.5 is not a contraindication to a neurosurgical procedure
- Platelet count greater than 70,000 is needed before a neurosurgical procedure
- Subcutaneous heparin and full anticoagulation should be avoided after ventriculostomy
- Prophylactic antibiotics or antibiotic-laced drains may prevent ventriculitis

---

Neurosurgical Emergencies by the Numbers

- ~80% of cerebellar hematomas develop acute hydrocephalus
- ~70% of epidural or subdural hematomas develop seizures
- ~50% of acute subdural hematomas also have contusions
- ~30% of cerebral hematomas further expand
- ~25% of traumatic contusions will deteriorate further
- ~10% of acute epidural hematomas are below tentorium

Putting It All Together

- Involve neurosurgeons early—waiting for deterioration may result in intervention coming too late
- Any patient with mass effect on CT scan deserves a neurosurgical opinion
- Decompressive craniectomy effectively treats increased intracranial pressure
- Few cerebellar hematomas can be managed medically
- Few contusions are managed surgically

References

1. Brown DL, Morgenstern LB. Stopping the bleeding in intracerebral hemorrhage. *N Engl J Med* 2005;352:828–830.
2. Byrne RW, Bagan BT, Bingaman W, Anderson VC, Selden NR. Emergency neurosurgical care solutions: acute care surgery, regionalization, and the neurosurgeon: results of the 2008 CNS consensus session. *Neurosurgery* 2011;68:1063–1067.
3. Byrne RW, Bagan BT, Slavin KV, et al. Neurosurgical emergency transfers to academic centers in Cook County: a prospective multicenter study. *Neurosurgery* 2008;62:709–716.
4. Cooper DJ, Rosenfeld JV, Murray L, et al. Decompressive craniectomy in diffuse traumatic brain injury. *N Engl J Med* 2011;364:1493–1502.
5. Felberg RA, Grotta JC, Shirzadi AL, et al. Cell death in experimental intracerebral hemorrhage: the "black hole" model of hemorrhagic damage. *Ann Neurol* 2002;51:517–524.
6. Garg RK, Liebling SM, Maas MB, et al. Blood pressure reduction, decreased diffusion on MRI, and outcomes after intracerebral hemorrhage. *Stroke* 2012;43:67–71.
7. Honeybul S, Ho KM, Lind CR, Gillett GR. The future of decompressive craniectomy for diffuse traumatic brain injury. *J Neurotrauma* 2011;28:2199–2200.
8. Kitaoka T, Hua Y, Xi G, Hoff JT, Keep RF. Delayed argatroban treatment reduces edema in a rat model of intracerebral hemorrhage. *Stroke* 2002;33:3012–3018.
9. Koeppen AH, Dickson AC, McEvoy JA. The cellular reactions to experimental intracerebral hemorrhage. *J Neurol Sci* 1995;134 Suppl: 102–112.
10. Lee KR, Betz AL, Keep RF, et al. Intracerebral infusion of thrombin as a cause of brain edema. *J Neurosurg* 1995;83:1045–1050.

11. Lee KR, Kawai N, Kim S, Sagher O, Hoff JT. Mechanisms of edema formation after intracerebral hemorrhage: effects of thrombin on cerebral blood flow, blood-brain barrier permeability, and cell survival in a rat model. *J Neurosurg* 1997;86:272–278.

12. Levin HS, Gary HE Jr, Eisenberg HM, et al. Neurobehavioral outcome 1 year after severe head injury: experience of the Traumatic Coma Data Bank. *J Neurosurg* 1990;73:699–709.

13. MacLellan CL, Auriat AM, McGie SC, et al. Gauging recovery after hemorrhagic stroke in rats: implications for cytoprotection studies. *J Cereb Blood Flow Metab* 2006;26:1031–1042.

14. MacLellan CL, Davies LM, Fingas MS, Colbourne F. The influence of hypothermia on outcome after intracerebral hemorrhage in rats. *Stroke* 2006;37:1266–1270.

15. MacLellan CL, Silasi G, Auriat AM, Colbourne F. Rodent models of intracerebral hemorrhage. *Stroke* 2010;41(10 Suppl):S95–S98.

16. Mayer SA, Lignelli A, Fink ME, et al. Perilesional blood flow and edema formation in acute intracerebral hemorrhage: a SPECT study. *Stroke* 1998;29:1791–9178.

17. Mendelow AD, Gregson BA, Fernandes HM, et al. Early surgery versus initial conservative treatment in patients with spontaneous supratentorial intracerebral haematomas in the International Surgical Trial in Intracerebral Haemorrhage (STICH): a randomized trial. *Lancet* 2005;365:387–397.

18. Mendelow AD, Gregson BA, Rowan EN, et al. Early surgery versus initial conservative treatment in patients with spontaneous supratentorial lobar intracerebral hematomas (STICH II): a randomized trial. *Lancet* 2013;382:397–408.

19. Nishino A, Suzuki M, Ohtani H, et al. Thrombin may contribute to the pathophysiology of central nervous system injury. *J Neurotrauma* 1993;10:167–179.

20. Petridis AK, Barth H, Buhl R, Hugo HH, Mehdorn HM. Outcome of cerebral amyloid angiopathic brain hemorrhage. *Acta Neurochir* 2008;150:889–895.

21. Polin RS, Shaffrey ME, Bogaev CA, et al. Decompressive bifrontal craniectomy in the treatment of severe refractory posttraumatic cerebral edema. *Neurosurgery* 1997;41:84–92.

22. Prabhakaran S, Gupta R, Ouyang B, et al. Acute brain infarcts after spontaneous intracerebral hemorrhage: a diffusion-weighted imaging study. *Stroke* 2010;41:89–94.

23. Prasad K, Mendelow AD, Gregson B. Surgery for primary supratentorial intracerebral hemorrhage. *Cochrane Database Syst Rev* 2008 4:CD000200.

24. Qureshi AI, Wilson DA, Traystman RJ. No evidence for an ischemic penumbra in massive experimental intracerebral hemorrhage. *Neurology* 1999;52:266–272.

25. Rabinstein AA, Atkinson JL, Wijdicks EFM. Emergency craniotomy in patients worsening due to expanded cerebral hematoma: to what purpose? *Neurology* 2002;58:1367–1372.

26. Rabinstein AA, Wijdicks EFM. Determinants of outcome in anticoagulation-associated cerebral hematoma requiring emergency evacuation. *Arch Neurol* 2007;64:203–206.

27. Rabinstein AA, Wijdicks EFM. Surgery for intracerebral hematoma: the search for the elusive right candidate. *Rev Neurol Dis* 2006;3:163–172.

28. Rodriguez-Luna D, Rubiera M, Ribo M, et al. Ultraearly hematoma growth predicts poor outcome after acute intracerebral hemorrhage. *Neurology* 2011;77:1599–1604.

29. Skriver EB, Olsen TS. Tissue damage at computed tomography following resolution of intracerebral hematomas. *Acta Radiol Diagn* 1986;27:495–500.

30. Sobani ZA, Shamim MS, Zafar SN, et al. Cranioplasty after decompressive craniectomy: An institutional audit and analysis of factors related to complications. *Surg Neurol Int* 2011;2:123.

31. Tanaka A, Yoshinaga S, Nakayama Y, Kimura M, Tomonaga M. Cerebral blood flow and clinical outcome in patients with thalamic hemorrhage: a comparison with putaminal hemorrhage. *J Neurol Sci* 1996;144:191–197.

32. Timmons SD, Ullman JS, Eisenberg HM. Craniectomy in diffuse traumatic brain injury. *N Engl J Med* 2011;365:373.

33. Walcott BP, Kwon CS, Sheth SA, et al. Predictors of cranioplasty complications in stroke and trauma patients. *J Neurosurg* 2013;118:757–762.

34. Wen L, Wang H, Wang F, et al. A prospective study of early versus late craniectomy after traumatic brain injury. *Brain Inj* 2011;25:1318–1324.
35. Xi G, Hua Y, Bhasin RR, Ennis SR, Keep RF, Hoff JT. Mechanisms of edema formation after intracerebral hemorrhage: effects of extravasated red blood cells on blood flow and blood-brain barrier integrity. *Stroke* 2001;32:2932–2938.
36. Xi G, Keep RF, Hoff JT. Mechanisms of brain injury after intracerebral haemorrhage. *Lancet Neurol* 2006;5:53–63.
37. Zazulia AR, Diringer MN, Videen TO, et al. Hypoperfusion without ischemia surrounding acute intracerebral hemorrhage. *J Cereb Blood Flow Metab* 2001;21:804–810.

7

Endovascular Options in Ischemic Stroke

If there is no collateral circulation of importance, an acute cerebral artery occlusion causes ischemia and necrosis of neural tissues. An intervention that restores circulation often limits damage, but not always, given that ischemic thresholds vary. The slogan "time is brain" does not apply to all patients— infarcts appear despite early reopening.[20,22,45] The decision concerning who would best benefit from such an intervention largely determines transfer of patients to certain centers.

Frustratingly, early treatment of a major stroke is full of uncertainty. If time allows—in essence 3 to 4.5 hours after onset—intravenous thrombolysis with tissue plasminogen activator (tPA or alteplase) is the first-line treatment for acute ischemic stroke.[3,20,43,53,56] Improvement after IV tPA administration can be immediate and even complete; but in many patients, the neurologic impairment may remain substantial or even worsen during infusion. Generally speaking, IV tPA is not a perfect drug, with recanalization in less than 50% and much less in acute proximal arterial occlusions.[38]

Therefore, in this day and age, acute effective treatment for major disabling stroke should involve sophisticated neuroimaging and endovascular options. Typically this is seen in patients with a severe incapacitating neurologic deficit. There is usually neurologic and radiological evidence of a large intracranial or extracranial vessel occlusion, or both. If a CT or MRI perfusion scan is available, the presence of a radiological penumbra suggests salvageable tissue, indicating he need for an endovascular approach straightaway.[60] These interventions usually come after IV tPA has "failed"—a debatable determinant. In patients with contraindications for intravenous thrombolysis, endovascular recanalization is promptly considered such as in patients with recent major surgeries, recent history of intracranial hemorrhage, or more obvious, time of symptom onset greater than 4.5 hours.[5]

It is self-evident that endovascular treatment—to advance microcathethers for intraarterial thrombolysis or to insert thrombectomy devices—has been a paradigm change in acute intervention of ischemic stroke.[27,31] Such a modern approach also involves significant resources and includes a cerebral angiogram team with anesthesiology support, an immediately available neurointerventionalist, and an expert in acute stroke management or a neurointensivist.[58] This field remains in flux and clinical approaches are modified often.[44]

Even if these resources are available, at what point during the assessment of the patient are these intervention teams sent for; and what could cause delay? What clinical and radiological metrics are used to determine eligibility? How are patients best managed after an intervention? This chapter reviews the selection of options for patients with acute ischemic stroke.

Principles

Current knowledge on endovascular treatment in the setting of an evolving stroke is based on several principles. This knowledge has been acquired over many years and has been extrapolated from clinical experience with large numbers of patients.

The first core principle is to reduce time before intervention as much as is feasible. Generally, the success of revascularization therapy may be related to the time of restoration of flow from the onset of symptoms. Clinical trials—testing intravenously administered thrombolytics—have found that the benefit is almost twice as high if the patient is treated within the first 90 minutes as compared to thrombolysis between 3 and 4½ hours. Intraarterial recanalization studies found that every 30-minute delay to recanalization was followed by 20% fewer patients achieving a good outcome.[30]

But there is more to it. Larger clots are more difficult to remove. Using intravenous thrombolytics for clots is often more successful in the distal middle cerebral artery branch than in the proximal middle cerebral artery or carotid artery occlusions. One can imagine that a large clot that is lodged in a large cerebral artery needs a physical pull or local delivery of a thrombolytic drug right inside the clot to dissolve the thrombus. Perhaps these distal branch occlusions are already broken-up clots that disintegrate more easily with intravenous thrombolytics. Still, nothing is absolute, because in acute carotid cervical occlusion, 50% of patients treated with intravenous tPA responded favorably. Good collateral flow in acute cervical internal carotid occlusion improved the probability of good outcome.[47] Distal carotid occlusions (so-called carotid T-occlusions) have a worse outcome due to poor collateral flow.

Here, tPA works when a higher concentration exceeds the inhibitors of tPA such as PAI-1. Clot characteristics also may play a role in whether recanalization may occur, though other factors may enter the equation. Clots ejected into the cerebral circulation are usually a mix of red (erythrocytes predominant) and white clots (platelets predominant). Most of the cardiac thrombi are red clots (red blood cells and fibrin) and do not contain calcifications and, therefore, should respond well to thrombolytic agents. To illustrate this further, cardiologists have been treating intracardiac clots with thrombolytic drug infusions for years with good results. White clots contain platelets, are not dissolved by thrombolytic agents, and are typically formed on pathologic endothelium or abnormal valves. Nonetheless, some have found that there is much less probability of clot lysis with intravenous thrombolytics in patients with known atrial fibrillation.[48] In this situation, a large clot burden is the likely explanation.[9,34]

A second core principle is that a patient presenting with a National Institutes of Health Stroke Scale (NIHSS) score greater than 10 increases the likelihood that a clot has to be treated with an endovascular approach.[19] Large deficits seen within an hour after onset rarely improve spontaneously or with intravenous thrombolysis. In some patients a so-called rapid shrinking deficit may occur, but there are no clinical or radiological characteristics that could set these patients apart. Most of the time, patients will continue to show a flaccid hemiparesis with forced eye deviation and neglect or global aphasia, depending on the involved hemisphere.

A third core principle is that the initial findings on CT scan or the size of the infarct core on CT perfusion might play an important role in determining the clinical outcome and risk of reperfusion hemorrhage.[59] Before determining eligibility of endovascular treatment, certain CT scan criteria can possibly predict outcome after recanalization. One of the major tasks at hand is to determine as early as possible whether there is salvageable ischemic neuronal tissue. Recanalizing and reperfusing (i.e., flooding) a large infarcted territory could lead to reperfusion hemorrhage.

A scoring system can help in determining whether the patient is likely to have a poor outcome after intravenous tPA. Many combined clinical and radiological scoring systems include the presence or absence of a hyperdense cerebral artery sign, the prestroke modified Rankin scale, age, glucose level on admission, time to treatment of less than 2 hours, and high NIHSS scores. A patient with a major hypodensity (typically defined as more than one-third of the middle cerebral artery territory) on a baseline CT scan will not benefit from endovascular treatment. A hyperdense middle cerebral artery sign indicates a proximal thromboembolus within the MCA or M1 segment. This sign, with high specificity but poor sensitivity (seen in only 20%–50% of cases), is recognized by a clot with an attenuation value of 60–90 HU. A dot sign can also be found in a middle cerebral artery (Sylvian fissure), which indicates an occlusion in a branch of the MCA (M2, or M3 branch), but that is not typically an area where mechanical thrombolysis is possible. A hyperdense basilar artery sign is a often missed CT finding. The challenge here is to differentiate between a slightly calcified basilar artery and a true clot. A tip of the basilar artery clot may show as a hyperdensity inside the pentagonal cisterns and may be misread as a partial volume effect of the clivus (Chapter 10).

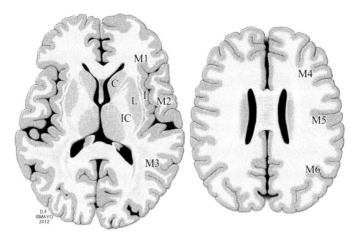

Figure 7.1 ASPECTS SCORE. For ASPECTS, the territory of the middle cerebral artery is allotted 10 points. 1 point is subtracted for an area of early ischemic change, such as focal swelling, or parenchymal hypoattenuation, for each of the defined regions. A normal CT scan has an ASPECTS value of 10 points. A score of 0 indicates diffuse ischemia throughout the territory of the middle cerebral artery. C = caudate; L = lentiform; IC = internal capsule; I = insular ribbon; MCA = middle cerebral artery; M1 = anterior MCA cortex; M2 = MCA cortex lateral to insular ribbon; M3 = posterior MCA cortex; M4, M5, and M6 are anterior, lateral, and posterior MCA territories immediately superior to M1, M2, and M3, rostral to basal ganglia. Subcortical structures are allotted 3 points (C, L, and IC). MCA cortex is allotted 7 points (I, M1, M2, M3, M4, M5, and M6).

One scoring system of particular interest is the Alberta Stroke Program Early CT Scan (ASPECTS) score. The ASPECTS score—starting at 10—subtracts one point for each area of hypoattenuation or loss of gray-white differentiation (Figure 7.1). It has been found that an ASPECTS score of <7 corresponds with a >70–100 mL infarct core and, thus, may be a cutoff of poor outcome. However, the interrater reliability of the ASPECTS score using this cutoff point is poor (weighted K of 0.53),[14] and a small caudate, lentiform nucleus, and insular infarct may already result in an ASPECTS score close to 7. It would be problematic to make decisions on endovascular approaches based on this score alone, but ASPECTS grading does bring the benefit of guiding physicians to look at CT scans in more detail. Moreover, it has become clear that involvement of neuroradiologists increases the reliability of the CT reading.[57]

A more sophisticated way of assessing pre-procedure status and risks of recanalization is to use contrast neuroimaging (perfusion CT or MRI). Areas of infarction can now be defined by restricted diffusion on the MRI scan; however, this modality is not available at all times and, thus, in many centers, decisions are currently based on a noncontrast CT scan followed by a CT angiogram and a CT scan perfusion.[15,16,18,42]

THE BASIC PRINCIPLES OF A PERFUSION CT SCAN

A perfusion CT scan requires a large-gauge catheter to allow rapid infusion of contrast. Placement of such a catheter alone may already delay the start of a CT perfusion and in some instances a catheter cannot be placed. Contrast is administered to patients who do not have a significantly increased serum creatinine, because the added risk of iodinated contrast nephrotoxicity is problematic. If contrast is needed, it is better used in one study and the cerebral angiogram. Obviously, perfusion CT scan has pitfalls, mostly technical. Every hospital with CT perfusion capabilities has experienced a learning curve with delays at multiple stops along the way.

The perfusion CT parameters that are used are cerebral blood volume (CBV), cerebral blood flow (CBF), mean transit time (MTT), and time to peak enhancement (TTP).[2,33,35,41] After injection of contrast, MTT is the time it takes for the contrast to pass through a given volume of brain. MTT is thus CBV/CBF. TTP is the time from the start of the contrast injection to maximal enhancement on CT.

How is CT perfusion interpreted? It is important to find matched (same area) or mismatched (not exactly the same area) perfusion abnormalities (Figure 7.2). The interpretation of a matched or nonmatched area is difficult for the untrained

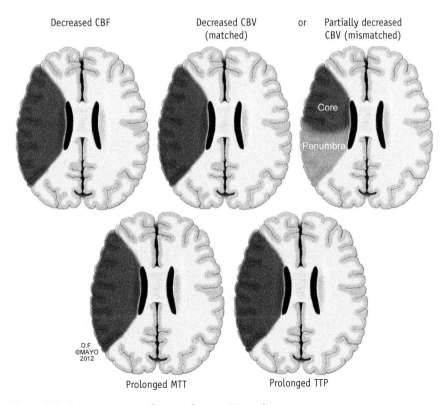

Figure 7.2 Determination of penumbra on CT perfusion scans.

eye. Opinions may vary on how much volume can be allowed to still fall into the matched category. In published series with large experience, it is roughly 50/50 match versus mismatch.[26] A matched perfusion abnormality between CBF and MTT or CBV maps indicates nonsalvageable brain tissue and has also been designated as "core infarct." (Usually seen as black areas, hence the expression "black won't come back.") Areas where there is prolonged MTT, reduced CBF, but normal CBV are interpreted as "ischemic penumbra." This assumes that compensatory mechanisms will preserve CBV in viable tissue. Such a penumbra may also be dependent on collateral flow, admission glucose level, hematocrit level, and blood pressure.[32,39]

If an MRI is available, a mismatch is usually assessed by evaluating CBF and diffusion-weighted imaging mismatch on a perfusion MRI.[52] Important insights recently came with serial MRI's scans before and after endovascular intervention. Failure to find a mismatch correlated strongly with worse outcome after reperfusion treatments.[26]

For many decades, ischemic stroke has been defined as a core of injury on its way to infarction but with penumbral areas that are potentially salvageable and could recover with the appropriate treatment.[17] Penumbra has always been described as certain CBF thresholds that are required for the preservation and function of normal brain tissue structure. The penumbra has been defined as an initially electrically silent area, and will improve or even completely restore if the CBF improves. There has also always been an understanding that the penumbra could progress into the infarct core if no action is taken.[21,24] Molecular correlates of such a penumbra have also been described and include decreased protein synthesis (but also still-preserved ATP synthesis of heat shock proteins) and unfolding protein response. The understanding has been that if these criteria were met, blood flow could be restored.[49] A recent discovery was that decrease in protein synthesis in the ischemic core results from unfolding protein response within the endoplasmic reticulum.[46] One concept is that the discontinuation of protein synthesis is a protective response to prevent formation of improperly processed proteins.[8] There is also experimental data showing that in the so-called infarct core there are multiple pockets of penumbra, also known as minipenumbras inside minicores (Figure 7.3). This is also supported by MRI scans that have shown that reduced apparent diffusion coefficient values in a low-CBF environment may improve if reperfusion occurs.[35] The new concept of minipenumbras in minicores has immediate clinical implications and points to the need for very early intervention to avoid minipenumbras blending into the minicores. Others have argued that a spreading depression wave is a major phenomenon in acute ischemia, a wave of cortical depolarization associated with collapse of ion pumps and impaired ATP generation, which may provide further insight in evolving ischemia.[54]

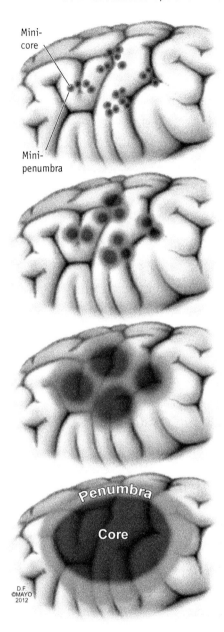

Figure 7.3 Minipenumbras evolving into large penumbra.

In Practice

One approach to treating patients with a large hemispheric stroke is shown in Tables 7.1 and 7.2. The first priority pertains to assessment of the clinical syndrome. Any large territorial involvement of the middle cerebral artery (MCA; M1 or stem occlusion) leads to early forced eye gaze toward the lesion, hemianopsia, hemiplegia of arm and leg (with some retained movement), neglect, or aphasia, depending on the affected hemisphere.[40] Ptosis may be very prominent in ischemia of the nondominant hemisphere. Occlusion of the superior trunk of the MCA produces a similar clinical picture. Occlusion of the inferior trunk of the MCA produces a Wernicke's aphasia when the dominant hemisphere is involved. Smaller territories such as a striatocapsular infarct (as a result of good collateral circulation) do produce a hemiplegia without sensory findings. Any early pupillary asymmetry (i.e., miosis) may be due to a Horner syndrome from acute carotid occlusion (thrombotic or dissection). Approximately 12 distal MCA branches can produce motor aphasias and abnormalities in spatial visual neglect. Pure motor hemiparesis with dysarthria points toward a lacunar syndrome possibly not eligible for endovascular treatment. The clinician therefore has the challenge—and obligation—of localizing the lesion. Unless the clinical findings are not particularly disabling, it is ill advised to exclude patients from further contrast imaging on the basis of clinical findings. Fluctuating clinical signs may indicate a large vessel occlusion and thus—perhaps paradoxically—should be imaged.

The distinctive clinical features of a major stroke in the anterior cerebral circulation are much less apparent in the posterior circulation.[29] Strokes in the posterior circulation are often not even considered by nonexperts. There are clearly clinical signs that are "unusual." Reduced consciousness due to involvement of the paramedian tegmental gray matter as part of the ascending reticular activating system is common in acute basilar artery occlusion, but nonspecific. Dysarthria, dysphagia, and horizontal gaze paresis are earlier presentations. An embolus at the top of the basilar artery may even present with more puzzling clinical signs

Table 7.1 **Principles for Triage to Endovascular Management**

- CT normal or only striatocapsular hypodensity
- IV tPA administration
- CT perfusion/CTA or MRI-DWI
- Determine core of infarcts (100 mL or not)
- Determine NIHSS sum score (20 or less)
- Window of intervention:
  - <8 hours anterior circulation
  - <24 hours posterior circulation
- Age (<80 years) and no major comorbidity and good life expectancy

Table 7.2 **Conditions to Be Met by Candidates for Endovascular Recanalization Therapy in Acute Ischemic Stroke**

- Severe, incapacitating neurologic deficits
- Large intracranial vessel occlusion
- Presence of radiological penumbra
- Failure of intravenous thrombolysis
  or
  Contraindications for intravenous thrombolysis, such as:
  - Time from symptom onset >4.5 hours
  - Recent surgery
  - History of intracranial hemorrhage
  - Active anticoagulation
- Good prestroke level of function
- Good rehabilitation potential

such as agitation (thalamus), cortical blindness (occipital involvement), sudden quadriplegia (base of the pons), and gaze-evoked nystagmus (cerebellum). Many patients with midbasilar or top-of-the-basilar clot may have shown early signs of vertigo, vomiting, abnormal gait, or even hemiparesis, only to deteriorate again with acute deep coma, loss of brainstem reflexes (fixed mid-position mesencephalic or pontine), acute bilateral internuclear ophthalmoplegia—found after cold water testing of the oculovestibular reflexes—and often extensor responses with additional limb jerks ("brainstem convulsions"). It is very difficult to exclude an acute basilar occlusion with certainty, and therefore CTA is more commonly obtained if clinical findings point toward the posterior circulation. CT perfusion of the pons, thalamus, and cerebellum is notoriously unreliable; decisions here are purely based on CTA findings.

The second priority pertains to assessment of the potential use of thrombolysis. The therapeutic window has been defined as 3 hours for IV thrombolysis (4.5 hours in ages <80), 6 hours for intraarterial thrombolysis of the anterior circulation, and 12 hours for intraarterial thrombolysis of the posterior circulation.

A recent large series of basilar artery occlusion treated patients with IV thrombolysis up to 48 hours after onset with good outcome in 50% suggests that IV tPA should be administered in many patients before cerebral angiogram.[51] Whether age should play a role in treatment of endovascular therapy is uncertain, but many experts feel that endovascular therapy in patients older than 80 years does not dramatically impact outcome.[25,56] Whether to proceed in this age group obviously also relates to the patients' comorbidity and functionality. When considering options one should always realize that patients with recanalization have a better chance of recovery than patients without recanalization.[10,38]

Suppose all options are on the table. In general, endovascular recanalization is considered when there is a major intracranial vessel occlusion.[1,6,23] This pertains to a clot location in the MCA M1 or proximal M2 (sylvian fissure) branch. In a patient with a distal M2 branch occlusion, intraarterial tPA may still be very beneficial, with an improvement in outcome. It is unclear whether M3 branches or insular branches should be treated aggressively with thrombolytics.

In the posterior circulation, endovascular treatment involves the basilar artery and the branching with the posterior cerebral artery. Endovascular treatment should only be considered if there is CT evidence of an ischemic penumbra with more than 25% mismatch between the area of perfusion abnormality and the area of reduced blood volume. When both a large territorial infarction and large penumbra are present, recanalization may not lead to better outcome. If there are large areas of infarction, postprocedural symptomatic hemorrhage might be quite likely—seen in 50% to 80% of patients after endovascular treatment.[6] In these situations it is therefore justified to not go beyond the initial treatment with IV tPA and take a loss.

The most difficult decision involves patients who present with a proximal artery occlusion (M1; M2; mid- and top-of-the-basilar artery), and on CT or MR perfusion show a major mismatch, but improve substantially or completely before a cerebral angiogram is started. Some of these patients may suddenly worsen hours later and develop a completed stroke. This is so frustrating that there is a good argument to be made to still recanalize these patients despite initial clinical improvement to avoid a sudden stroke from happening later. Many experts in this field would favor such an aggressive approach, but there is no proven benefit.

Mechanical clot disruption can be performed with several devices and this innovative field is rapidly evolving. So far, three devices have been used. The first was the MERCI device, which pierces the thrombus and uses microwires to remove the clot.[4,50,51] Next came mechanical thrombectomy with a thrombus aspiration (PENUMBRA™) device.[36,37] These are microcatheters advanced to the surface of the clot, with suction force applied. Small catheters may even enter M2 segments. Most recently used are self-expandable stent thrombectomy devices, and the largest trial has been performed with the SOLITAIRE™.[7] Two recent clinical trials showed stent retrievers are superior to MERCI retriever with regard to reperfusion.[6] These devices are shown in Figure 7.4. Feasibility studies have shown that use of any of these devices can result in rapid restoration of flow. There will be a plethora of new devices.

The modern treatment of acute stroke may evolve into intravenous thrombolysis immediately followed by retrieval.[4,13,28,31,55] However, the use of intraarterial thrombolysis has significantly increased recanalization rate—to approximately 60% partial or complete recanalization.[27] Combining intraarterial thrombolysis with mechanical fragmentation may even increase recanalization rates to 80%. The degree of recanalization is, however, variable and may be partly successful rather than complete in a third of patients.

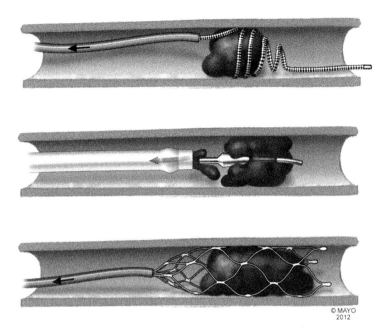

Figure 7.4 Endovascular Devices (cork screw, suction, and stent retrieval).

The thrombolysis in cerebral infarction (TICI) classification, which has been validated, is simple and can be helpful in classifying results of the intervention (Table 7.3).[61] Prognosis after endovascular treatment may be related to site of the obstruction, clinical presentation, and whether recanalization has been established. Postprocedure neuroimaging may not be necessarily predictive unless

Table 7.3 **TICI Reperfusion Scale**

mTICI Grades	Definitions
Grade 0	No perfusion
Grade 1	Antegrade reperfusion past the initial occlusion, but limited distal branch filling with little or slow distal reperfusion
Grade 2a	Antegrade reperfusion of less than half of the occluded target artery previously ischemic territory (eg. in 1 major division of the MCA and its territory)
Grade 2b	Antegrade reperfusion of more than half of the previously occluded target artery ischemic territory (eg, in 2 major divisions of the MCA and their territories)
Grade 3	Complete antegrade reperfusion of the previously occluded target artery ischemic territory, with absence of visualized occlusion in all distal branches

MCA indicates middle cerebral artery; and mTICI, Modified Treatment in Cerebral Ischemia Scale.

Table 7.4 **Indicators of Poor Prognosis**

- Major clinical findings
- Lack of recanalization or persistent distal occlusion
- Coma with extensor posturing
- Large area of matching deficit on CT perfusion before the intervention
- Absence of large radiological penumbra before the intervention
- Poor collateral arterial supply
- Internal carotid artery occlusion
- Postprocedural intracranial hemorrhage

large territories or eloquent territories are infarcted. Some of the criteria for poor outcome are summarized in Table 7.4. Most recently several major clinical trials have compared endovascular treatment with IV tPA (MR-RESCUE) IV tpA and endovascular treatment compared with IV tPA (IMS III) and IV tpA to endovascular treatment (SYNTHESIS). All these trials found no benefit of endovascular treatment. These trials have been strongly criticized and editorialized.[37] Major misgivings include use of "obsolete" devices, inappropriate preoperative imaging and small number of patients per center among other concerns. Its effect on practice cannot be assessed at this time, but these results may reduce triage to endovascular treatment centers.

By the Way

- There are other modifiable factors (e.g., hyperglycemia, hypoxemia, hypotension)
- Major neurologic deficit may remain with little tissue loss of eloquent brain
- Stuttering signs may become major deficits
- When collaterals are poor resolving signs in a major vessel occlusion may still warrant clot retrieval
- Improvement may be delayed after recanalization

Endovascular Treatment for Stroke by the Numbers

- ~80% of patients with ischemic stroke treated with retrieval devices recanalize
- ~60% of patients with ischemic stroke treated with IA tPA recanalize
- ~30% of patients with ischemic stroke treated with IV tPA recanalize
- ~20% of patients with ischemic stroke are treated with IV tPA
- ~15% of patients with ischemic stroke eligible for endovascular treatment

Putting It All Together

- Window of opportunity closes quickly
- Neurointervention is likely needed with NIHSS of 10 or more
- CTA is considered when no improvement is seen 30 minutes after IV tPA infusion is completed or when symptoms fluctuate markedly
- CT or MRI perfusion identifies salvageable brain, core infarct, and risk of reperfusion
- Recanalization of a proximal clot is rarely spontaneous
- Use any available means to achieve recanalization

References

1. Alexandrov AV, Grotta JC. Arterial reocclusion in stroke patients treated with intravenous tissue plasminogen activator. *Neurology* 2002;59:862–867.
2. Allmendinger AM, Tang ER, Lui YW, Spektor V. Imaging of stroke: Part 1, Perfusion CT—overview of imaging technique, interpretation pearls, and common pitfalls. *AJR Am J Roentgenol* 2012;198:52–62.
3. Balami JS, Hadley G, Sutherland BA, Karbalai H, Buchan AM. The exact science of stroke thrombolysis and the quiet art of patient selection. *Brain* 2013;136:3528–3553.
4. Baker WL, Colby JA, Tongbram V, et al. Neurothrombectomy devices for the treatment of acute ischemic stroke: state of the evidence. *Ann Intern Med* 2011;154:243–252.
5. Brinjikji W, Rabinstein AA, Kallmes DF, Cloft HJ. Patient outcomes with endovascular embolectomy therapy for acute ischemic stroke: a study of the national inpatient sample: 2006 to 2008. *Stroke* 2011;42:1648–1652.
6. Broderick JP, Schroth G. What the SWIFT and TREVO II trials tell us about the role of endovascular therapy for acute stroke. *Stroke* 2013;44:1761–1764.
7. Castaño C, Dorado L, Guerrero C, et al. Mechanical thrombectomy with the Solitaire AB device in large artery occlusions of the anterior circulation: a pilot study. *Stroke* 2010;41:1836–1840.
8. Del Zoppo GJ, Sharp FR, Heiss WD, Albers GW. Heterogeneity in the penumbra. *J Cereb Blood Flow Metab* 2011;31:1836–1851.
9. Fredieu A, Duckwiler G, Starkman S, et al. Clot burden in acute ischemic stroke: relation to occlusion site and the success of revascularization therapy. *Stroke* 2005;36:449–450.
10. Furlan A, Higashida R, Wechsler L, et al. Intra-arterial prourokinase for acute ischemic stroke: the PROACT II study: a randomized controlled trial; prolyse in acute cerebral thromboembolism. *JAMA* 1999;282:2003–2011.
11. Furlan AJ. Clot retrieval for stroke should be restricted to clinical trials: no. *Stroke* 2010;41:194–195.
12. Gralla J, Brekenfeld C, Mordasini P, Schroth G. Mechanical thrombolysis and stenting in acute ischemic stroke. *Stroke* 2012;43:280–285.
13. Grotta JC, Welch KM, Fagan SC, et al. Clinical deterioration following improvement in the NINDS rt-PA Stroke Trial. *Stroke* 2001;32:661–668.
14. Gupta AC, Schaefer PW, Chaudry ZA, et al. Interobserver reliability of baseline noncontrast CT Alberta Stroke program early CT Score for intra-arterial stroke treatment selection. *Am J Neuroradiology AJNR* 2012;33:1046–1049.
15. Hacke W, Furlan AJ, Al-Rawi Y, et al. Intravenous desmoteplase in patients with acute ischemic stroke selected by MRI perfusion-diffusion weighted imaging or perfusion CT

(DIAS-2): a prospective, randomised, double-blind, placebo-controlled study. *Lancet Neurol* 2009;8:141–150.

16. Hallevi H, Barreto AD, Liebeskind DS, et al. Identifying patients at high risk for poor outcome after intra-arterial therapy for acute ischemic stroke. *Stroke* 2009;40:1780–1785.

17. Heiss WD. The ischemic penumbra: correlates in imaging and implications for treatment of ischemic stroke. The Johann Jacob Wepfer award 2011. *Cerebrovasc Dis* 2011;32:307–320.

18. Hopyan J, Ciarallo A, Dowlatshahi D, et al. Certainty of stroke diagnosis: incremental benefit with CT perfusion over noncontrast CT and CT angiography. *Radiology* 2010;255:142–153.

19. IMS II Trial Investigators. The Interventional Management of Stroke (IMS) II Study. *Stroke* 2007;38:2127–2135.

20. IMS Study Investigators. Combined intravenous and intra-arterial recanalization for acute ischemic stroke: the Interventional Management of Stroke Study. *Stroke* 2004;35:904–911.

21. Kanekar SG, Zacharia T, Roller R. Imaging of stroke: Part 2. Pathophysiology at the molecular and cellular levels and corresponding imaging changes. *AJR Am J Roentgenol* 2012;198:63–74.

22. Khatri P, Abruzzo T, Yeatts SD, et al. Good clinical outcome after ischemic stroke with successful revascularization is time-dependent. *Neurology* 2009;73:1066–1072.

23. Khatri P, Hill MD, Palesch YY, et al. Methodology of the Interventional Management of Stroke III trial. *Int J Stroke* 2008;3:130–137.

24. Kidwell CS, Alger JR, Saver JL. Beyond mismatch: evolving paradigms in imaging the ischemic penumbra with multimodal magnetic resonance imaging. *Stroke* 2003;34:2729–2735.

25. Kim D, Ford GA, Kidwell CS, et al. Intra-arterial thrombolysis for acute stroke in patients 80 and older: a comparison of results in patients younger than 80 years. *AJNR Am J Neuroradiol* 2007;28:159–163.

26. Lansberg MG, Straka M, Kemp S, et al. MRI profile and response to endovascular reperfusion after stroke (DEFUSE 2): a prospective cohort study. *Lancet Neurol* 2012;11:860–867.

27. Lee M, Hong KS, Saver JL. Efficacy of intra-arterial fibrinolysis for acute ischemic stroke: meta-analysis of randomized controlled trials. *Stroke* 2010;41:932–937.

28. Levy EI, Siddiqui AH, Crumlish A, et al. First Food and Drug Administration approved prospective trial of primary intracranial stenting for acute stroke: SARIS (stent-assisted recanalization in acute ischemic stroke). *Stroke* 2009;40:3552–3556.

29. Mattle HP, Arnold M, Lindsberg PJ, Schonewille WJ, Schroth G. Basilar artery occlusion. *Lancet Neurol* 2011;10:1002–1014.

30. Mazighi M, Serfaty JM, Labreuche J, et al. Comparison of intravenous alteplase with a combined intravenous-endovascular approach in patients with stroke and confirmed arterial occlusion (RECANALISE study): a prospective cohort study. *Lancet Neurol* 2009;8:802–809.

31. Meyers PM, Schumacher HC, Connolly ES Jr, et al. Current status of endovascular stroke treatment. *Circulation* 2011;123:2591–2601.

32. Natarajan SK, Dandona P, Karmon Y, et al. Prediction of adverse outcomes by blood glucose level after endovascular therapy for acute ischemic stroke. *J Neurosurg* 2011;114:1785–1799.

33. Obach V, Oleaga L, Urra X, et al. Multimodal CT-assisted thrombolysis in patients with acute stroke: a cohort study. *Stroke* 2011;42:1129–1131.

34. Ogata J, Yutani C, Otsubu R, et al. Heart and vessel pathology underlying brain infarction in 142 stroke patients. *Ann Neurol* 2008;63:770–781.

35. Olivot JM, Mlynash M, Thijs VN, et al. Relationships between cerebral perfusion and reversibility of acute diffusion lesions in DEFUSE: insights from RADAR. *Stroke* 2009;40:1692–1697.

36. Penumbra Pivotal Stroke Trial Investigators. The Penumbra Pivotal Stroke Trial: safety and effectiveness of a new generation of mechanical devices for clot removal in intracranial large vessel occlusive disease. *Stroke* 2009;40:2761–2768.

37. Pierot L, Gralla J, Cognard C, White P. Mechanical thrombectomy after IMS III, synthesis, and MR-RESCUE. *AJNR Am J Neuroradiol* 2013;34:1671–1673.

38. Rha JH, Saver JL. The impact of recanalization on ischemic stroke outcome: a meta-analysis. *Stroke* 2007;38:967–973.

39. Ribo M, Molina C, Montaner J, et al. Acute hyperglycemia state is associated with lower tPA-induced recanalization rates in stroke patients. *Stroke* 2005;36:1705–1709.
40. Ropper AH, Shafran B. Brain edema after stroke. Clinical syndrome and intracranial pressure. *Arch Neurol* 1984;41:26–29.
41. Rostrup E, Knudsen GM, Law I, et al. The relationship between cerebral blood flow and volume in humans. *Neuroimage* 2005;24:1–11.
42. Röther J. Imaging-guided extension of the time window: ready for application in experienced stroke centers? *Stroke* 2003;34:575–583.
43. Saver JL, Fonarow GC, Smith EE, et al. Time to treatment with intravenous tissue plasminogen activator and outcome from acute ischemic stroke. *JAMA*. 2013;309:2480–2488.
44. Saver JL. The evolution of technology. *Stroke* 2013;6 Suppl 1:S13–S15.
45. Saver JL. Improving reperfusion therapy for acute ischaemic stroke. *J Thromb Haemost* 2011;9:333–343.
46. Schröder M, Kaufman RJ. The mammalian unfolded protein response. *Annu Rev Biochem* 2005;74:739–789.
47. Seet RCS, Wijdicks EFM, Rabinstein AA. Acute stroke from cervical internal carotid artery occlusion: treatment results and predictors of outcome. *Arch Neurol* 2012;24:1–6.
48. Seet RCS, Zhang Y, Wijdicks EFM et al. Relationship between chronic atrial fibrillation and worse outcome in stroke patients after intravenous thrombolysis. *Arch Neurol* 2011;68:1454–1458.
49. Sharp FR, Lu A, Tang Y, Millhorn DE. Multiple molecular penumbras after focal cerebral ischemia. *J Cereb Blood Flow Metab* 2000;20:1011–1032.
50. Smith WS, Sung G, Saver J, et al. Mechanical thrombectomy for acute ischemic stroke: final results of the multi MERCI trial. *Stroke* 2008;39:1205–1212.
51. Strbian D, Sairanen T, Silvennoinen H, et al. Thrombolysis of basilar artery occlusion: Impact of baseline ischemia and time. *Ann Neurol* 2013;73:688–694.
52. Souza LC, Yoo AJ, Chaudhry ZA, et al. Malignant CTA collateral profile is highly specific for large admission DWI infarct core and poor outcome in acute stroke. *AJNR Am J Neuroradiol* 2012;33:1331–1336.
53. Strbian D, Meretoja A, Ahlhelm FJ, et al. Predicting outcome of IV thrombolysis-treated ischemic stroke patients: The DRAGON score. *Neurology* 2012;78:427–432.
54. Strong AJ. Spreading depolarizations: tsunamis in the injured brain. *Adv Clin Neurosci Rehab* 2009;9:32–35.
55. Sung SM, Lee TH, Cho HJ, et al. Recanalization with wingspan stent for acute middle cerebral artery occlusion in failure or contraindication to intravenous thrombolysis: a feasibility study. *AJNR Am J Neuroradiol* 2012;33:1156–1161.
56. The IST-3 collaborative group, Sandercock P, Wardlaw JM, et al. The benefits and harms of intravenous thrombolysis with recombinant tissue plasminogen activator within 6 h of acute ischemic stroke (the third international stroke trial [IST-3]): a randomized controlled trial. *Lancet* 2012;379:2352–2363.
57. Wardlaw JM, Von Kummer R, Farrall AJ, et al. A large web-based observer reliability study of early ischemic signs on computed tomography: the Acute Stroke Cerebral CT Evaluation of Stroke Study (ACCESS) *PlosOne* 2010;5:e15757.
58. Wintermark M, Albers GW, Alexandrov AV, et al. Acute stroke imaging research roadmap. *Stroke* 2008;39:1621–1628.
59. Wintermark M, Meuli R, Browaeys P, et al. Comparison of CT perfusion and angiography and MRI in selecting stroke patients for acute treatment. *Neurology* 2007;68:694–697.
60. Yoo AJ, Pulli B, Gonzalez RG. Imaging-based treatment selection for intravenous and intra-arterial stroke therapies: a comprehensive review. *Expert Rev Cardiovasc Ther* 2011;9:857–876.
61. Zaidat OO, Yoo AJ, Khatri P, et al. Recommendations on angiographic revascularization grading standards for acute ischemic stroke: a consensus statement. *Stroke* 2013;44:2650–2663.

8

Supporting Acute Respiratory
Muscle Weakness

Neuromuscular respiratory failure is usually part of an already established neurologic disorder, a consequence of the natural progression of the disorder and rarely a presenting feature. For the uninitiated physician, acute respiratory failure may seem like a new problem, but when, for example, signs of myasthenia gravis (MG) or amyotrophic lateral sclerosis (ALS) become apparent, there must have been somewhere a delay or misdiagnosis.[12,13] Once it becomes clear that the patient has a manageable neurologic disorder, a concentrated effort is required to treat it appropriately.

There are difficult decisions to be made after assessment of the nature of respiratory failure. These are: triage of the patient, how to instruct the nursing staff to recognize worsening, and what set of tests to order that could assist in both the diagnosis and in anticipating serious problems down the line.

Patients with acute neuromuscular respiratory failure are often less prudently judged, and every year patients "code on the floor," often at night. In every instance, after careful review, warning signs were present that could have prompted a better triage—preferably to a monitored setting.

How do we best test for neuromuscular respiratory failure, and what is the basic pathophysiology? How do we choose the most appropriate mode of ventilation? When is a tracheostomy warranted? These are some of the questions that will be answered in this chapter.

Principles

The clinical presentation of air hunger and rapid shallow breathing due to a fatiguing respiratory muscle pump—leading to low arterial PO_2 and high arterial PCO_2—can be understood as an interplay of factors. This section reviews respiratory mechanics and when abnormal how they change clinical presentation and laboratory tests.

RESPIRATORY PUMP FAILURE

During respiration, lungs can expand and recoil in two ways: by downward and upward movement of the diaphragm that lengthens and shortens the chest cavity, and by elevation and depression of the ribs to increase and decrease the anteroposterior diameter of the chest. Normal quiet breathing is largely accomplished by contraction of the diaphragm. In general, the diaphragm is responsible for approximately two-thirds of ventilatory effort to generate inspiration. It may be supplemented by accessory inspiratory muscles including the external intercostals, scalene, and sternocleidomastoid muscles. Expiration is usually due to recoil of the thoracic cage, but abdominal wall muscles may also be necessary to generate expiration and are responsible for a forceful cough. Generally the pressure generated by the diaphragm is dependent on its three-dimensional shape, but it is also dependent on Laplace's law, which implies an inverse relationship between radius and pressure: shortening increases pressure.

Although the upper airway muscles do not contribute directly to chest expansion, they are essential for keeping the airways open during respiration. They play an important role in preventing collapse of the pharynx during inspiration and preventing aspiration during swallowing.

What might also be relevant here is whether the muscle fibers are fast- or slow-twitch types. With the exception of laryngeal muscles, oropharyngeal muscles have a higher proportion of fast fibers. Their weakness can therefore be seen early on in acute neuromuscular disorders because slow fibers have a higher fatigue resistance than fast fibers due to their high oxidative metabolism.[52] The diaphragm, on the other hand, has an equal proportion of slow and fast muscle fibers, which—in association with small fiber size and large number of capillaries—makes it more resistant to fatigue.[55,58,64,65]

Another major component of breathing relates to the mechanics of the chest wall. A large muscle plate such as the diaphragm is necessary to bring a significant change in lung volume. During contraction, there is a tilting and flattening of the diaphragm in the anterior/posterior direction. Such a movement has been compared with a piston in a cylinder; but because of associated ribcage expansion, it is most like a piston in an expanding cylinder. Function of the diaphragm is also affected by intraabdominal pressure (such as in a traumatic abdominal compartment syndrome), and it is also affected by the chest wall elasticity (e.g., advanced Parkinson's disease). Most commonly, marked obesity (more specifically a "pot belly") may result in intraabdominal hypertension in a supine position, creating a cranial shift of the diaphragm and increased pleural pressure. All of it will increase the work of breathing.

Moving air into the lungs is dependent on respiratory load (the sum of resistance of inspiratory flow, the resistance of the chest wall and lungs, and the positive pressure at peak expiration). When inspiratory muscles contract, a negative force overcomes this respiratory load, resulting in inward movement of air. With weakness, the respiratory load can only be partly overcome, leading to less airflow and to collapse of lung areas. Compliance is the willingness of the lung to distend; its measurement is determined by the change in volume divided by change in pressure (C = $\Delta V/\Delta P$). The inverse of compliance is elastance, defined as the willingness of the lung to return to a resting position. Neuromuscular weakness is basically a decreased interthoracic compliance; maximal inspiratory flow is limited by muscle strength and the poor compliance of the lung and chest wall.

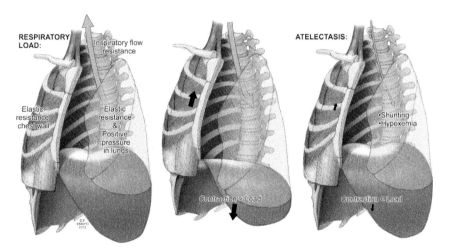

Figure 8.1 Consequences of increased inspiratory load and diaphragmatic weakness.

The neuromuscular respiratory failure thus follows a predictable pattern: failure of diaphragm and intercostal muscles followed by compensatory use of accessory muscles, eventually resulting in hypoventilation and atelectasis, further leading to shunting and hypoxia[72] (Figure 8.1). Whether long-standing poor mechanics lead to microatelectasis is unclear, but it seems to be much less of an issue in patients with chronic neuromuscular disorders.[23]

Weakness of respiratory muscles causes low tidal volume ("shallow") breathing and poor gas exchange, leading to tachypnea and later hypercapnia.[59] These patients also have increased dead space ventilation next to their elevated respiratory drive. The rapid breathing is the result of signals to the respiratory center from the abnormal and weak respiratory muscle. Usually the arterial PCO_2 will decrease due to this rapid breathing; but when respiratory muscle strength is more than 25% of normal, PCO_2 will increase.[46]

The ventilatory drive's response to climbing PCO_2 remains intact.[18-20,59] In more chronic neuromuscular disorders, this response is "blunted," meaning there is no appropriate response to increased PCO_2. The ventilatory drive response to

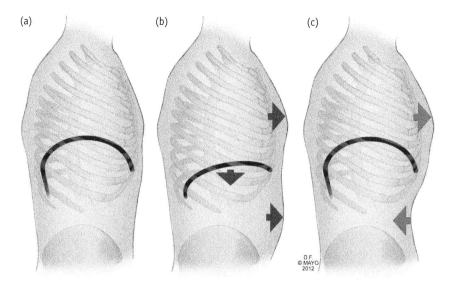

Figure 8.2 Normal breathing excursions (a,b). Paradoxical breathing due to diaphragm failure (c).

an acute increase in $PaCO_2$ in patients with Guillain-Barré syndrome (GBS) and myasthenia gravis (MG) remains.[6,32,50]

The first indication of diaphragmatic weakness is alveolar hypoventilation and impaired CO_2 exchange.[37,41,45,47] Alveolar hypoventilation may also become more apparent with sleep or when the patient performs a simple exercise. These changes are followed by an increase in respiratory rate as a compensatory mechanism to maintain minute ventilation. Later, accessory muscles of ventilation are recruited in response to increased ventilatory demand. Paradoxical breathing, also known as thoracoabdominal asynchrony, occurs with severe respiratory muscle weakness. Normally, the abdomen and chest expand and contract in a synchronized fashion. During inspiration, a downward movement of the diaphragm pushes the abdominal contents down and out as the rib margins are lifted and moved out, causing both chest and abdomen to rise.[1] With diaphragmatic weakness or paralysis, the diaphragm moves up rather than down during inspiration and the abdomen moves in, contracting during chest rise. (A video showing these features has been published recently).[72]

During speaking, the patient will pause frequently but breathlessness improves in upright position.[4,26,28,29] Oropharyngeal muscle weakness results in threatening collapse of upper airway musculature. Furthermore, coughing—deep inspiration and closure of glottis and contraction of abdominal muscles—is understandably weak, could eventually lead to aspiration, and could further worsen the hypoxia.

RESPIRATORY PUMP FAILURE ASSESSED WITH
LABORATORY TESTS

Phrenic nerve stimulation can be used to asses the function of the diaphragm.[16,43,44,54] The phrenic nerve is located underneath the posterior border of the sternocleidomastoid muscle and can easily be stimulated with a surface electrode. Electrical stimuli of 0.05- to 0.2-ms duration will produce a diaphragmatic muscle compound action potential. Repetitive nerve stimulation studies can also be performed in patients suspected of having MG or Lambert-Eaton syndrome. Testing is usually repeated, asking the patient to continuously inspire through an incentive spirometer for 10 seconds. Phrenic nerve stimulation might be diagnostic and can help in differentiating among myopathy, myasthenic syndrome, acute neuropathy, and chronic neuropathy. It is self-evident that phrenic nerve conduction alone is not sufficient, and needle EMG must be performed. Needle EMG of the diaphragm provides evidence of denervation and may show low amplitudes of the motor action potential, but also large motor units indicating a chronic denervation as typically seen in ALS. The risk of pneumothorax is very low and has been found to be 2/1,000 procedures (Figure 8.3). Phrenic nerve stimulation might be diagnostic and can help in differentiating among myopathy, myasthenic syndrome, acute neuropathy, and chronic neuropathy. These tests are mainly diagnostic. Denervation of the diaphragm muscle does not necessarily predict failure to wean from ventilatory support. Phrenic nerve and diaphragmatic studies have no predictive value for future intubation or need for respiratory support and do not predict length of recovery time. The patterns of abnormalities in phrenic nerve conduction and needle EMG are identical to other muscle disorders.

Generally, electrophysiological studies will suggest the cause of respiratory failure, and criteria have been well established. Electrodiagnostic criteria for a demyelination is compound muscle action potential amplitude less than 50%, conduction velocity less than 75% of normal, and distal latency more than 130% of normal—all reflecting abnormal stimulus propagation along the nerve fibers. When conduction fails in several fibers, the amplitude decreases and is named conduction block if the amplitudes of distal and proximal stimulation sites are different. Conduction block, A waves, and dispersed (spread out) F waves are the first abnormalities. Demyelinating disorders also lack fibrillation potentials and sharp waves. In a neuromuscular transmission defect, there will be an increase in the latency of the diaphragm compound muscle action potential, a decrease in amplitude, normal morphology, and decreased motor unit potentials.[24] In myopathies there is normal diaphragm compound muscle action potential and amplitude. The motor unit potentials in myopathies are decreased in number, and the morphology is abnormal.

Neuromuscular weakness of the respiratory muscles is characterized by the inability to generate or maintain normal respiratory pressures. The degree of

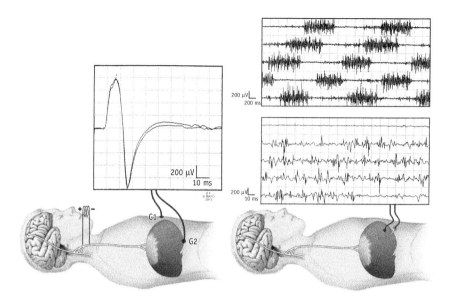

Figure 8.3 Phrenic nerve conduction and EMG of diaphragm (motor unit potentials at different sweeps).

involvement of the inspiratory and expiratory muscles is variable, but the clinical manifestations reflect the compromise of both muscle groups. Ventilation remains intact until diaphragm involvement becomes significant.

Pulmonary function tests are most important in assessing diaphragmatic function and respiratory muscle strength, usually involving vital capacity, maximal inspiratory pressure (MIP), and maximal expiratory pressure (MEP).[14,17,42,33,51] Pulmonary studies typically reveal a pure ventilatory defect with otherwise normal pulmonary parenchyma. The ventilatory defect may worsen with development of atelectasis.

Respiratory muscle force examination is dependent on several factors.[5,10,27] First, position with patients who lean forward generate higher inspiratory pressures, and patients in recumbent position generate lower inspiratory pressures.[2] Second, leaks are common when there is pressure generation in the muscles of the cheek and buccal muscles. Usually the MEP is twice the MIP and when the MEP is less than the MIP it is often due to leaks. Some patients suck on buccal muscles and do not generate sufficient pressures. This can be prevented by placement of a scuba device. Third, several repetitions are needed to come to a valid and reliable measurement. In general, a minimum of three measurements should be performed, showing a variance less than 10%. All these measurements are volitional and therefore may be effort dependent. If all three test results are similarly normal or decreased, it is more likely that it represents a maximal effort by the patient.

In patients with diaphragmatic weakness, the vital capacity falls when the patient is supine and it must decrease by more than 25% to be called abnormal. A high MIP (>80 cm water), particularly in combination with a normal vital capacity, makes a neuromuscular respiratory failure unlikely.[63]

Questionable efforts could be followed up by a sniff nasal pressure maneuver. The sniff maneuver is more useful because it is more natural and easier for the patient to understand. Several studies have found that the test is quite useful in acute neuromuscular disease, but it may be inferior to more traditional methods in more severe neuromuscular disorders.[35] Sniff pressures, in which pressure is measured in the esophagus during a sniff, may be more reliable although this requires a more standardized setting, usually in a pulmonary function laboratory and therefore is not practical at the bedside.[25,36,66,68] The sniff maneuver might also be hindered by insufficient nasal passages in some patients.[15]

In more slowly progressive neurologic disorders, these pulmonary function tests are also important because—for example—a normal MIP or MEP in ALS indicates that the patient may likely be spared mechanical ventilation in 6 months. The MEP >60 cm water may also predict the ability to cough in patients with neuromuscular disease, and in one study, a MEP >70 cm water also was correlated with a >50% predictive value of tracheostomy-free survival.[62] This, again, emphasizes the importance of a good expiratory pressure and the ability to cough effectively, which reduces the chance of mucus plugging and pneumonia.

Pulse oximetry is important in any patient with neuromuscular respiratory disease, but obviously it does not identify CO_2 retention. Rapid and shallow breathing leads to chronic hypercapnia in patients with neuromuscular disease. With rapid, shallow breathing the total volume is markedly decreased, the inspiratory time is shortened, and vital capacity is truncated, resulting in hypercarbia. Nevertheless, overnight pulse oximetry is useful because nocturnal hypoventilation indicates respiratory muscle weakness in the appropriate setting.[70]

Arterial blood gas measurements can be informative, but also may not be. It may show a hypoxemic hypercapnic respiratory failure in a patient in obvious respiratory distress. However, in more subtle presentations the arterial blood gas can be deceptively normal even in a markedly fatigued patient. Normally one would expect a reduced $PaCO_2$ in a tachypneic patient. A normal arterial PCO_2 in a tachypneic patient therefore is a sign of pending fatigue because, as a result of mechanical failure, the patient cannot "blow off" CO_2. In other words, poor bellows lead to poor ventilation due to alveolar collapse, resulting in hypoxemia. There is a "normal" $PaCO_2$, which only rises when there is complete system failure.

In Practice

There are difficulties and limitations in recognition of acute neuromuscular respiratory failure. There are several caveats that should be known: (1) it will be very difficult to be completely certain the patient will oxygenate well enough; (2) pulmonary function tests can be unreliable due not only to poor patient effort but also to ineffective coaching; (3) failure to manage secretions, as simple as it is, with the addition of respiratory muscle weakness, may be the most common reason for acute intubation; (4) normal blood gases are not necessarily reassuring and may even precede respiratory arrest; and (5) the degree of limb weakness does not always coincide with involvement of the diaphragm. In other words, upper arm weakness may be absent in failing diaphragm function.

Furthermore, a minority of patients with acute neuromuscular weakness may have an unusual medical condition, and it should be considered if there are atypical presentations. These are highly uncommon, but because treatment is different they need to be excluded quickly: severe thyrotoxicosis, hypermagnesemia, hypophosphatemia (often seen as a result of refeeding syndrome), hypokalemia and hyperkalemia in extreme forms may all cause weakness and respiratory failure and can be recognized by laboratory tests (Table 8.1).

Another common problem is evaluating a critically ill patient for neurologic disease when it has become abundantly clear that weaning is not only prolonged but appears to be impossible. The damage that mechanical ventilation can cause is substantial, and diaphragmatic weakness may already occur at the end of the first week of ventilation.[38] Diaphragm dysfunction (and evolving atrophy) may occur in approximately 30% of critically ill patients when assessed with ultrasonography.[39] The challenge here is to distinguish respiratory muscle failure due to critical illness from acute or subacute neurologic disease.[21] Typical neurologic findings that are worrisome are: atrophy, fasciculations (ALS), myotonia and weakness

Table 8.1 **Uncommon Causes for Respiratory Failure and Acute Weakness**

- Tick paralysis
- Botulism
- Organophosphate poisoning
- Fish poisoning (tetrodotoxin)
- Snake bite
- Vasculitis
- Hypophosphatemia
- Hypokalemia/hyperkalemia
- Hypermagnesemia
- Acute porphyria

(myotonic dystrophy), jaw and neck muscle weakness, ophthalmoplegia and ptosis (MG) or a sensory level and long tract signs (spinal cord lesion).

Respiratory failure is most frequently seen in GBS and MG, and eventually always in progressive neuromuscular disorders. Respiratory failure is common in congenital myasthenic syndromes, and many children eventually require a permanent tracheostomy.

Respiratory failure in MG is also difficult to recognize. Patients may have incrementally been increasing their cholinesterase inhibitors (by themselves or after physician's advice) and may have excessive salivation and sweating, abdominal cramps, and urinary urgency. MG associated with muscle specific tyrosine kinase (MuSK) antibodies do have more prominent oculobulbar weakness, although they develop more generalized weakness eventually.[30,31] Patients with MuSK antibody–positive MG have much less successful response to acetylcholine esterase inhibitors.[8]

Respiratory failure and GBS can be assessed clinically, as with any other case of acute neuromuscular respiratory failure. Several studies have found that vital capacity and proximal distal compound muscle action potential ratio of the common perineal nerve are independent predictors of mechanical ventilation and disability.[22]

Others found that the time between onset of weakness and hospital admission, the presence of facial weakness or oropharyngeal dysfunction, and the severity of limb weakness assessed by the medical research council subscore predicted respiratory failure and intubation. This confirms the clinical impression that difficulty clearing secretions in patients with a rapid onset, defined as 3 days after onset, may indicate a high likelihood of intubation.[69]

Intubation in neuromuscular disorders may have some risks due to use of drugs administered during rapid-sequence intubation. Most known is the exaggerated hyperkalemia response with succinylcholine in chronic neuromuscular diseases. This response is due to an up-regulation of receptors but it may also be associated with rhabdomyolysis. Patients with myotonic dystrophy and Becker's myopathy are at highest risk, but the whole phenomenon remains uncommon. If a patient with myasthenia gravis is intubated, nondepolarizing neuromuscular blocking agents are preferred due to increased sensitivity in these patients as a result of destruction of acetylcholine receptors.[11] This effect can be more profound if patients were already treated with a high dose of pyridostigmine.[49] Therefore, it is common practice to proceed with a reduced dose of rocuronium 0.9 to 1.2 mg/kg for rapid sequence intubation, and to avoid succinylcholine.

RESPIRATORY ASSISTANCE

As a general rule, imminent neuromuscular respiratory failure is typically recognized by restlessness, tachycardia with a rate of >100 per minute, tachypnea

with a respiratory rate of >20 per minute, use of sternocleidomastoid or scalene muscles, constantly interrupting speech to catch a breath, asynchronous
breathing and sometimes paradoxical breathing, and the presence of forehead
sweating. It should be pointed out that patients will continue to have a sensation of breathlessness even in the presence of normal blood gas. When $PaCO_2$
rises, patients will then experience "air hunger," which is a result of increase in
respiratory drive and a result of a hypercapnic stimulation of chemoreceptors.
The sensation of hypoxemia can be different, however, and patients will develop
a sensation of "rapid breathing." Patients often struggle to breathe indicating
that intubation is necessary. Noninvasive ventilation (biphasic positive airway
pressure or BiPAP) may be a first choice in MG and is occasionally successful.[53]
BiPAP is not a good option in GBS. Unfortunately intubation and mechanical
ventilation is a common pathway in these two disorders.

Noninvasive ventilation is also usually a first option in patients presenting in
respiratory failure from ALS. The indications are a combination of clinical findings (orthopnea, nocturnal awakening) and pulmonary pressures (usually less
than 50% of predicted). Noninvasive mechanical ventilation reduces the work
of breathing, may reverse hypercapnia, and reverses atelectasis. Mucolytics are
needed (anticholinergics), and sometimes botulinum toxin injections into the
salivary glands in patients with severe bulbar weakness. Settings are simple and
at the lowest level possible, usually 10–12 cm water for inspiratory positive airway pressure and 5–6 cm water for expiratory pressure to allow for CO_2 blow-off.
The arterial blood gas guides the adjustment of the settings of BiPAP. Hypercapnia
may be chronic and may not lower too much with BiPAP. In many patients with
bulbar dysfunction, a tracheostomy is needed and is found acceptable by quite a
few patients with ALS.

WEANING FROM RESPIRATORY ASSISTANCE

Any patient that has been ventilated for a prolonged period of time will need
a plan for weaning from the ventilator.[67] Unfortunately, once patients with
ALS are intubated, it is highly unlikely they can be liberated from the ventilator, except for a few who may be treated with BiPAP alone.[60] Generally
weaning from mechanical ventilation should be guided by improvement in
strength and normalization of values on serial pulmonary function tests. In
GBS, diaphragmatic weakness may reverse before extremity weakness; thus,
the timing of weaning should not be gauged solely by recovery of extremity
muscle strength.

There are several conditions that need to be considered before attempting
to wean the patient from the ventilator. In myasthenia gravis, one important

priority is to have satisfactory treatment of the myasthenic symptoms. In addition, the patient should have no major pulmonary problems, no evidence of atelectasis, pleural effusions, or have marked difficulty handling secretions. Secretion volume, determining whether the patient is comfortable with a T-piece trial, and normal chest X-ray all have a good predictive value for successful extubation in any patient with acute neuromuscular respiratory failure. Pulmonary function tests can in some sense predict weaning but are far from reliable. The MEP, which reflects coughing up of secretions and thus recovering abdominal musculature strength, might be the best predictor of successful weaning.

In GBS, weaning from mechanical ventilation should be undertaken as early as possible because of the number of significant complications related to prolonged mechanical ventilation. However, one should anticipate weeks on the ventilator. The weaning process can be initiated once vital capacity (VC) reaches 25 mL/kg and spontaneous tidal volumes of 10 to 12 mL/kg are attained. MIP exceeding –50 cm water and VC improvement by 4 mL/kg from preintubation to preextubation are also associated with successful extubation. Reducing intermittent mandatory ventilation rate or reducing pressure support level can be used as a weaning protocol.

In MG weaning from the mechanical ventilator may be initiated early. An optimal dose of pyridostigmine needs to be found, and patients will not likely be able to be liberated from the ventilator without adequate treatment even after multiple administration IV immunoglobulin (IVIG) or plasma exchange courses.[7,9]

The weaning process in patients with MG often is challenging because of the fluctuating nature of the disease. Reintubation is not uncommon.[61] In selected patients, noninvasive ventilation can be used for bridging during the weaning process to prevent reintubation. Older age, pneumonia, and atelectasis are major risk factors for extubation failure.

In MG weaning trials may begin when VC exceeds 15 mL/kg, MIP exceeds –30 cm water, and oxygenation is adequate on inspired oxygen concentrations (FiO$_2$) of 40% or less. It is important to reintroduce cholinesterase inhibitors before extubation trials are initiated. Weaning methods may vary. Patients can be switched to continuous positive airway pressure (CPAP) with pressure support ventilation (PSV). A decrease in tidal volume and increases in respiratory and heart rates are indicators of fatigue. Once the patient demonstrates good endurance at low pressure support (5 cm water), usually for more than 2 hours, extubation can be considered, but often T-piece trials are needed first. After extubation, incentive spirometry is helpful to reduce the risk of atelectasis and reintubation.

SPECIFIC TREATMENT AND OTHER CONCERNS

Treatment for GBS is plasma exchange or IVIG, but treatment for MG involves corticosteroids and plasma exchange or IVIG.[40] Plasma exchange may involve 5 to 7 exchanges of 2 to 3 liters each, usually every other day. In MG, plasma exchange markedly reduces autoantibodies, and there is clinical improvement both in patients with acetylcholine receptor antibodies as well as patients with MuSK antibodies. Patients with anti-MuSK antibodies plasma exchange is the preferred treatment, but in more resistant patients rituximab has been administered.[34] In a newly diagnosed MG, thymectomy may be considered but this procedure may have to be postponed because surgery can itself worsen myasthenia or cause a new crisis.[48]

Specific treatment for GBS or MG may cause complications. Treatment with IVIG can be associated with acute renal disease due to its high sucrose load and may significantly worsen in susceptible patients and lead to a marked rise in creatinine, even up to a point that dialysis is temporarily needed (sucrose light IVIG may prevent that—e.g., Gamunex®).

Finally, it is also important to recognize that acute neuromuscular disease has autonomic effects, with potential systemic complications. Many patients with severe GBS will have dysautonomia, manifested by cardiac arrhythmias and wide blood pressure swings. Dysautonomia may potentially contribute to severe hypotension during introduction of positive pressure ventilation. MG has been associated with significant hypothyroidism and needs to be recognized. Autoimmune thyroid diseases such as Hashimoto's thyroiditis and Graves disease do occur in approximately 10% of patients with MG and require detailed testing. Patients with chronic neuromuscular disorders, particularly patients with MG or chronic inflammatory demyelinating polyneuropathy (CIDP), may have developed chronic effects of immunosuppression, including type 2 diabetes mellitus, obesity, osteoporosis, and renal disease.

By the Way

- Early neuromuscular respiratory failure presents with frequent pauses during sentences and shortness of breath with supine position
- Hypoxemia comes before hypercarbia
- Arterial blood gas can be normal in neuromuscular respiratory failure
- Electrophysiological tests and pulmonary function tests are diagnostic but not predictive of need for mechanical ventilation

---

Neuromuscular Respiratory Failure by the Numbers

- 90% need for tracheostomy with respiratory failure and GBS
- 60% need for tracheostomy with respiratory failure and MG
- 50% reduction in pulmonary function requires intubation in acute disease
- 30% of patients with MG require reintubation after initial weaning
- 20% of patients with GBS require respiratory support

Putting It All Together

- Rapid shallow breathing with marginal oxygenation typifies diaphragmatic weakness
- Atelectasis results in hypoxemia then results in hypercarbia, then may result in respiratory arrest
- BiPAP is ideal for MG and ALS
- In MG, weaning from the ventilator—once intubated—is difficult to predict and erratic
- Immunomodulating therapy is needed in GBS and MG, but will not prevent intubation in most of the patients

References

1. Alexander C. Diaphragm movements and the diagnosis of diaphragmatic paralysis. *Clin Radiol* 1966;17:79–83.
2. Allen SM, Hunt B, Green M. Fall in vital capacity with posture. *Br J Dis Chest* 1985;79:267–271.
3. Alshekhlee A, Miles JD, Katirji B, Preston DC, Kaminski HJ. Incidence and mortality rates of myasthenia gravis and myasthenic crisis in US hospitals. *Neurology* 2009;72:1548–1554.
4. American Thoracic Society. Dyspnea. Mechanisms, assessment, and management: a consensus statement. *Am J Respir Crit Care Med* 1999;159:321–340.
5. American Thoracic Society/European Respiratory Society. ATS/ERS Statement on respiratory muscle testing. *Am J Respir Crit Care Med* 2002;166:518–624.
6. Annane D, Quera-Salva MA, Lofaso F, et al. Mechanisms underlying effects of nocturnal ventilation on daytime blood gases in neuromuscular diseases. *Eur Respir J* 1999;13:157–162.
7. Barth D, Nabavi Nouri M, Ng E, Nwe P, Bril V. Comparison of IVIg and PLEX in patients with myasthenia gravis. *Neurology* 2011;76:2017–2023.
8. Benatar M. A systematic review of diagnostic studies in myasthenia gravis. *Neuromuscul Disord* 2006;16:459–467.
9. Berrousch OTJ, Baumann I, Kalischewski P, et al. Therapy of myasthenia crisis. *Crit Care Medicine* 1997;25:1228–1235.
10. Black LF, Hyatt RE. Maximal respiratory pressures: normal values and relationship to age and sex. *Am Rev Respir Dis* 1969;99:696–702.

11. Blichfeldt-Lauridsen L, Hansen BD. Anesthesia and myasthenia gravis. *Acta Anaesthesiol Scand* 2012;56:17–22.

12. Bolton CF, Chen R, Wijdicks EFM, Zifko UA. *Neurology of Breathing*. Amsterdam, Elsevier, 2004.

13. Burakgazi AZ, Höke A. Respiratory muscle weakness in peripheral neuropathies. *J Peripher Nerv Syst* 2010;15:307–313.

14. Cabrera Serrano M, Rabinstein AA. Usefulness of pulmonary function tests and blood gases in acute neuromuscular respiratory failure. *Eur J Neurol* 2012;19:452–456.

15. Chaudri MB, Liu C, Watson L, Jefferson D, Kinnear WJ. Sniff nasal inspiratory pressure as a marker of respiratory function in motor neuron disease. *Eur Respir J* 2000;15:539–542.

16. Chen R, Collins S, Remtulla H, Parkes A, Bolton CF. Phrenic nerve conduction study in normal subjects. *Muscle Nerve* 1995;18:330–335.

17. Demedts M, Beckers J, Rochette F, Bulcke J. Pulmonary function in moderate neuromuscular disease without respiratory complaints. *Eur J Respir Dis* 1982;63:62–67.

18. Derenne JP, Macklem PT, Roussos C. The respiratory muscles: mechanics, control, and pathophysiology. *Am Rev Respir Dis* 1978;118:119–133.

19. Derenne JP, Macklem PT, Roussos C. The respiratory muscles: Mechanics, control, and pathophysiology. Part 2. *Am Rev Respir Dis* 1978;118:373–390.

20. Derenne JP, Macklem PT, Roussos C. The respiratory muscles: mechanics, control, and pathophysiology. Part III. *Am Rev Respir Dis* 1978;118:581–601.

21. Doorduin J, van Hees HW, van der Hoeven JG, Heunks LM. Monitoring of the respiratory muscles in the critically ill. *Am J Respir Crit Care Med* 2013;187:20–27.

22. Durand MC, Porcher R, Orlikowski D, et al. Clinical and electrophysiological predictors of respiratory failure in Guillain-Barré syndrome: a prospective study. *Lancet Neurol* 2006;5:1021–1028.

23. Estenne M, Gevenois PA, Kinnear W, et al. Lung volume restriction in patients with chronic respiratory muscle weakness: the role of microatelectasis. *Thorax* 1993;48:698–701.

24. Farrugia ME, Vincent A. Autoimmune mediated neuromuscular junction defects. *Curr Opin Neurol* 2010;23:489–495.

25. Fitting JW, Paillex R, Hirt L, Aebischer P, Schluep M. Sniff nasal pressure: a sensitive respiratory test to assess progression of amyotrophic lateral sclerosis. *Ann Neurol* 1999;46:887–893.

26. Galtrey CM, Faulkner M, Wren DR. How it feels to experience three different causes of respiratory failure. *Pract Neurol* 2012;12:49–54.

27. Gibson GJ, Pride NB, Davis JN, Loh LC. Pulmonary mechanics in patients with respiratory muscle weakness. *Am Rev Respir Dis* 1977;115:389–395.

28. Gibson GJ. Diaphragmatic paresis: pathophysiology, clinical features, and investigation. *Thorax* 1989;44:960–970.

29. Griggs RC, Donohoe KM, Utell MJ, Goldblatt D, Moxley RT 3rd. Evaluation of pulmonary function in neuromuscular disease. *Arch Neurol* 1981;38:9–12.

30. Guptill JT, Sanders DB, Evoli A. Anti-MuSK antibody myasthenia gravis: clinical findings and response to treatment in two large cohorts. *Muscle Nerve* 2011;44:36–40.

31. Guptill JT, Sanders DB. Update on muscle-specific tyrosine kinase antibody positive myasthenia gravis. *Curr Opin Neurol* 2010;23:530–535.

32. Guz A. Brain, breathing and breathlessness. *Respir Physiol* 1997;109:197–204.

33. Hamnegård CH, Wragg S, Kyroussis D, et al. Portable measurement of maximum mouth pressures. *Eur Respir J* 1994;7:398–401.

34. Hart IK, Sharshar T, Sathasivam S. Immunosuppressive drugs for myasthenia gravis. *J Neurol Neurosurg Psychiatry* 2009;80:5–6.

35. Hart N, Polkey MI, Sharshar T, et al. Limitations of sniff nasal pressure in patients with severe neuromuscular weakness. *J Neurol Neurosurg Psychiatry* 2003;74:1685–1687.

36. Héritier F, Rahm F, Pasche P, Fitting JW. Sniff nasal inspiratory pressure. A noninvasive assessment of inspiratory muscle strength. *Am J Respir Crit Care Med* 1994;150:1678–1683.

37. Hutchinson D, Whyte K. Neuromuscular disease and respiratory failure. *Pract Neurol* 2008;8:229–237.
38. Jaber S, Petrof BJ, Jung B, et al. Rapidly progressive diaphragmatic weakness and injury during mechanical ventilation in humans. *Am J Respir Crit Care Med* 2011;183:364–371.
39. Kim WY, Suh HJ, Hong SB, Koh Y, Lim CM. Diaphragm dysfunction assessed by ultrasonography: influence on weaning from mechanical ventilation. *Crit Care Med* 2011;39:2627–2630.
40. Lacomis D. Myasthenia crisis. *Neurocrit Care* 2004;3:189–194.
41. Laghi F, Tobin MJ. Disorders of the respiratory muscles. *Am J Respir Crit Care Med* 2003;168:10–48.
42. Leech JA, Ghezzo H, Stevens D, Becklake MR. Respiratory pressures and function in young adults. *Am Rev Respir Dis* 1983;128:17–23.
43. Mier A, Brophy C, Moxham J, Green M. Phrenic nerve stimulation in normal subjects and in patients with diaphragmatic weakness. *Thorax* 1987;42:885–888.
44. Mier A, Brophy C, Moxham J, Green M. Repetitive stimulation of phrenic nerves in myasthenia gravis. *Thorax* 1992;47:640–644.
45. Mier-Jedrzejowicz A, Brophy C, Moxham J, Green M. Assessment of diaphragm weakness. *Am Rev Respir Dis* 1988;137:877–883.
46. Misuri G, Lanini B, Gigliotti F, et al. Mechanism of CO_2 retention in patients with neuromuscular disease. *Chest* 2000;117:447–453.
47. Moxham J. Respiratory muscle fatigue: mechanisms, evaluation and therapy. *Br J Anaesth* 1990;65:43–53.
48. Nam T-S, Lee S-H, Kim B-C, et al. Clinical characteristics and predictive factors of myasthenic crisis after thymectomy. *J Clin Neurosci* 2011;18:1185–1188.
49. Nilsson E, Meretoja OA. Vecuronium dose-response and maintenance requirements in patients with myasthenia gravis. *Anesthesiology* 1990;73:28–32.
50. Panitch HB. Diurnal hypercapnia in patients with neuromuscular disease. *Paediatr Respir Rev* 2010;11:3–8.
51. Polkey MI, Green M, Moxham J. Measurement of respiratory muscle strength. *Thorax* 1995;50:1131–1135.
52. Polla B, D'Antona G, Bottinelli R, Reggiani C. Respiratory muscle fibres: specialisation and plasticity. *Thorax* 2004;59:808–817.
53. Rabinstein AA, Wijdicks EFM. BiPAP in acute respiratory failure due to myasthenia crisis may prevent intubation. *Neurology* 2002;59:1647–1649.
54. Resman-Gaspersc A, Podnar S. Phrenic nerve conduction studies: technical aspects and normative data. *Muscle Nerve* 2008;37:36–41.
55. Roussos C, Macklem PT. The respiratory muscles. *N Engl J Med* 1982;307:786–797.
56. Roussos C, Zakynthinos S. Fatigue of the respiratory muscles. *Intensive Care Med* 1996;22:134–155.
57. Roussos C. Function and fatigue of respiratory muscles. *Chest* 1985;88:124S–132S.
58. Roussos C. The failing ventilatory pump. *Lung* 1982;160:59–84.
59. Roussos C. Ventilatory muscle fatigue governs breathing frequency. *Bull Eur Physiopathol Respir* 1984;20:445–451.
60. Schmidt EP, Drachman DB, Wiener CM, et al. Pulmonary predictors of survival in amyotrophic lateral sclerosis: use in clinical trial design. *Muscle Nerve* 2006;33:127–132.
61. Seneviratne J, Mandrekar J, Wijdicks EFM, Rabinstein AA. Predictors of extubation failure in myasthenia gravis. *Arch Neurol* 2008;65:929–933.
62. Simon PM, Schwartzstein RM, Weiss JW, et al. Distinguishable types of dyspnea in patients with shortness of breath. *Am Rev Respir Dis* 1990;142:1009–1014.
63. Terzi N, Orlikowski D, Fermanian C, et al. Measuring inspiratory muscle strength in neuromuscular disease: one test or two? *Eur Respir J* 2008;31:93–98.
64. Tobin MJ, Chadha TS, Jenouri G, Birch SJ, Gazeroglu HB, Sackner MA. Breathing patterns, 2. Diseased subjects. *Chest* 1983;84:286–294.
65. Tobin MJ, Chadha TS, Jenouri G, Birch SJ, Gazeroglu HB, Sackner MA. Breathing patterns, 1. Normal subjects. *Chest* 1983;84:202–205.

66. Uldry C, Fitting JW. Maximal values of sniff nasal inspiratory pressure in healthy subjects. *Thorax* 1995;50:371–375.
67. Vassilakopoulos T, Zakynthinos S, Roussos Ch. Respiratory muscles and weaning failure. *Eur Respir J* 1996;9:2383–2400.
68. Verin E, Delafosse C, Straus C, et al. Effects of muscle group recruitment on sniff transdiaphragmatic pressure and its components. *Eur J Appl Physiol* 2001;85:593–598.
69. Walgaard C, Lingsma HF, Ruts L, et al. Prediction of respiratory insufficiency in Guillain-Barré syndrome. *Ann Neurol* 2010;67:781–787.
70. White JE, Drinnan MJ, Smithson AJ, Griffiths CJ, Gibson GJ. Respiratory muscle activity and oxygenation during sleep in patients with muscle weakness. *Eur Respir J* 1995;8:807–814.
71. Wijdicks EFM. Short of breath, short of air, short of mechanics. *Pract Neurol* 2002;2:208–213.
72. Wijdicks EFM. Neurogenic paradoxical breathing. *J Neurol Neurosurg Psychiatry* 2013; 84:1296.

9

Emergencies in the Transplant Recipient

Organ transplantation remains a taxing surgical procedure and a daunting prospect for patients. Nevertheless, a large number of patients go through transplantation successfully. The early phase (<60 days) may include prolonged intensive care admission, and this is particularly true for patients with heart-lung and combined organ transplants and certainly after bone marrow transplantation. The risk for a critical illness is markedly increased, and patients who may seem to be doing remarkably well may have a quick setback. Generally speaking, any patients with a recent solid organ or hematopoietic stem cell transplantation may develop graft-versus-host disease, multiorgan failure, and shock. In these sicker patients, neurologic complications are very possible. The later phase (60–365 days) after transplantation includes proclivity for infections and much later—although it may be only a few months—secondary malignancies may appear. Most impressive is post-transplant lymphoproliferative disease (PTLD), likely explained by the introduction of genetic material of an Epstein-Barr virus (EBV) seropositive donor into an EBV seronegative recipient.

A transplant recipient who develops an acute neurologic disorder poses an immediate challenge for consultants, not least in examining a critically ill patient with polypharmacy. It requires specialized knowledge; the more traditional neurologic disorders are far less common, and "exotic causes" predominate (particularly when it comes to evaluation of stupor and fever). These patients may rapidly develop a fulminant medical and neurologic clinical course if the cause is not recognized and remediated.

Neurologic manifestations (or complications) are uncommon in renal transplantation but may reach a prevalence of 10%–20% in cardiac, liver, or lung transplantation.[2,3,6,16,28,35] Neurologic complications may result in an increased risk of early demise. Most instructively—when reviewed in more detail—the majority of patients with a lung transplantation were found to have a neurologic complication, with a third seriously affecting quality of life or causing a fatal outcome.[19] That leaves the question of whether neurologic complications are sufficiently recognized.

There are several other considerations. First, neurologic complications may be specific to the type of transplantation. Neurologic complications associated with bone marrow transplantation are quite different from those associated with transplantation of an organ such as a kidney or liver. Second, seizures are often drug-related and equally common as a result of permanent structural lesions. It is a difficult task to implicate certain drugs, but some commonly used drugs lower the seizure threshold. Third, any structural lesion in the brain may be due to infection and requires immediate treatment. Fourth, major sodium abnormalities and osmotic shifts can be seen after liver transplantation, causing osmotic demyelination.

Neurologists who provide consultative services to transplant recipients may only see a fraction of all postoperative problems, because many are handled by the transplant team. If they occur and are considered "out of the ordinary," a neurologic opinion is sought. Over the years, the complexity of these consults has increased, and neurologists suddenly may have to tackle a formidable problem. This is an area where one may find extremely difficult situations. What is the spectrum of abnormalities in a transplant recipient with an acute neurologic problem? How can we narrow down the differential diagnosis? Which patients are at high risk for complications, and how can a neurologist be useful? This chapter systematically discusses the major acute neurologic illnesses that have been recognized in the transplant recipient.

Principles

Knowledge about several core topics is needed to grapple with the neurologic complications of a recent transplant recipient. There are patterns, however, and brain injury after transplantation mostly comes from anoxic-ischemic injury, drug toxicity, or infections in these highly susceptible patients. A sudden intracranial hemorrhage is often a total surprise.

One principle is to judge neurologic complications in relation to the type of transplant. The risks to the central nervous system (CNS) are related to the extent of the operation, in much the same way as in any other major surgical procedure involving multiple vascular sutures and extracorporeal circulation.

Patients with cardiac or lung transplantation are at high risk of postoperative stroke due to hypotension and hypoxemia, and injury can be severe. In many of the patients, the first signs are of what appears as a poorly defined encephalopathy—in others, seizures are a presenting symptom.[11] Heart, lung, or combined heart-lung transplantation exposes the patient to complications of cannulation from placement of the cardiopulmonary bypass. Immediate—and very common—risks are bleeding, cardiac arrhythmias, or ventricular failure. Although brain injury may result from poor perfusion—as suggested by abnormalities in so called watershed areas—constant embolization is a far more likely mechanism. Cannulation of an atherosclerotic ascending aorta may be emboligenic, but dislodgement can also occur during the procedure if some of the catheters "powerwash" out mobile atherosclerotic debris. In many patients, prolonged hypotension cannot be easily implicated, except in situations with marked hypotension in patients temporarily placed on extra corporeal membrane oxygenation (ECMO). This procedure markedly increases the risk of anoxic-ischemic encephalopathy.

In lung transplantations, persistent hypotension may occur from right ventricular failure during intraoperative pulmonary artery clamping or as a result of fluid restriction (to avoid pulmonary edema in the postoperative phase).

Liver transplantation exposes the recipient to several risks. The pretransplant coagulopathy is worsened by frequent infusions of coagulation factors and antithrombotic agents, but surprisingly, the risk of intracerebral hemorrhage is not markedly increased in this phase. Intracranial pressure is normal in patients undergoing liver transplantation, except when an acutely necrotic liver is replaced. In some instances, a superior vena cava thrombosis at the side of the venous inflow of the venovenous bypass may suddenly increase backflow pressure and intracranial pressure. The procedure-related complications with pancreas or kidney (or combined) transplantation are no different from those of other major abdominal surgeries.

Another core principle is to understand the different types of immunosuppression. There has been a major transition from glucocorticoids and azathioprine to calcineurin inhibitors and mTOR inhibitors, each with a different side-effect profile and each with the potential for interfering with transplant pharmacopeia, which may increase levels and lead to toxicity.[10,32] Side effects of these drugs remain common and fortunately only lead to mild toxicity of immunosuppressive therapy.[22,30,33,35] Considering the large proportion of patients on immunosuppressive agents, neurotoxicity is quite uncommon. Often some sort of drug interference or drugs that increase the availability of this drug produces toxicity. These drugs are often antibiotics or antifungals such as erythromycin and fluconazole.

Cyclosporin and tacrolimus are both calcineurin inhibitors, but breakdown of the blood-brain barrier is still needed for these drugs to enter. Some other injury may have occurred that increases the likelihood of neurotoxicity (i.e., surgical hypotension or hypoxemia). These drugs bind to an immunophilin that blocks calcineurin. This protein is involved in self-signaling and maintenance of cytoskeletal protein function, that is to say inhibition of the protein triggers apoptosis pathways.

Other new immunosuppressive approaches with monoclonal antibodies targeting CD40 have not resulted in any early neurologic complications. B-cell depleting CD20 antibody rituximab is currently also of interest, but does not appear to result in any early neurologic complications. Figure 9.1 summarizes the T-cell targets of current immunosuppressants.

The hallmarks of a calcineurin inhibitor neurotoxicity are the development of bizarre behavior, psychosis, and hallucinations that are characteristically

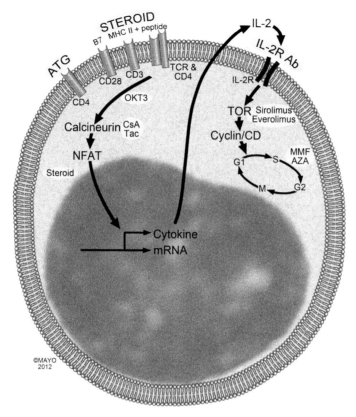

Figure 9.1 Current immunosuppressive agents and targets.
CDK: cyclin-dependent kinase; NFAT: nuclear factor of activated cells;
ATG: antithymocyte globulin; MHC: major histocompatibility complex; TCR: T-cell
receptor; IL2RAB: interleukin-2 receptor antibody; MMF: mycophenolate mofetil;
AZA: azathioprine.

vivid and visual with bright colors. Blindness, nonsensical speech, stuttering, or
becoming mute is seen in more extreme forms. Seizures often do occur, and status
epilepticus could appear in a matter of hours.

The CT scan may not be revealing, often showing dubious hypodensities that
are frequently misinterpreted as cerebral infarctions. An MRI scan will show
the significant areas of vasogenic edema, mostly in the occipital and parietal
regions, though they can also be in the thalamus or other locations in the CNS.
The abnormalities are very similar to posterior reversible encephalopathy syndrome (PRES). These abnormalities may occur directly as a neurotoxic effect but
later, when management of calcineurin-associated hypertension may become
more difficult to manage, hypertension may cause PRES in transplant recipients.

Discontinuation of the drug and replacement of a calcineurin inhibitor with siro-limus is the most effective treatment. Recovery, including awakening from coma, can be protracted.

A third principle to consider in evaluating transplant patients is the unusual spectrum of opportunistic infections.[21] Infections in transplant recipients can be categorized in three time periods. Infection disease experts have used the following time periods: the first month post transplantation, 6 months post transplantation, or more than 6 months after transplantation. These time periods do appear to contain certain risks for certain infections.[12,34] Gram-negative bacteria *Escherichia coli* or *Pseudomonas aeruginosa* may disseminate into the CNS, though only rarely.[26] In the immediate post-transplantation period, reactivation of a CNS viral infection is usually seen in bone marrow transplant recipients and often involves herpes viruses such as herpes simplex virus (HSV), varicella-zoster virus, and human herpesvirus 6 (HHV-6). All of these viruses can cause encephalitis, which may present with altered levels of consciousness and usually a confusional state and occasional focality, such as aphasia or hemiparesis. In the period of 2–6 months after transplantation, patients are at highest risk for more common known immunocompromised-related CNS infections. These infections are *Aspergillus* species, *Nocardia*, or *Toxoplasma gondii* and, in occasional patients, due to cytomegalovirus, HSV, HHV-6, and varicella-zoster virus. Each of these infections has a more or less typical presentation, summarized in Table 9.1 for consideration. Later infections, defined as after 6 months, are meningitis associated with *Cryptococcus neoformans*, *Histoplasma capsulatum*, or *Coccidioides immitis*, but each of these infections is region-specific. The most concerning late effect of long-term immunosuppression is the development of progressive multifocal leukoencephalopathy due to JC viral infection.[20] A rare complication of transplantation is EBV-associated PTLD. PTLD has been divided into several categories and progresses from plasmacytic hyperplasia to polymorphic, monomorphic, and classic Hodgkin lymphoma types. These lymphomas are more likely high grade and aggressive, with CNS involvement. Reduction of immunosuppression, rituximab, or anthracycline-based chemotherapy may lead to regression. Surveillance includes repeated EBV polymerase chain reaction (PCR) to monitor virus load.

In Practice

There are some general issues and more organ-specific problems. The most commonly encountered reason for a consultation or advice has to do with general assessment of an "altered state of consciousness." The appearance of a new encephalopathy may be due to rejection dysfunction of the graft, or may have other causes.

Table 9.1 **Central Nervous System Infections in Transplant Recipients**

Organism	Time from TX (months)	Presentation	CT or MRI	CSF	Diagnosis
Listeria monocytogenes	1–6	Headache, stupor (prior abdominal cramps and diarrhea)	Meningeal enhancement only; brainstem involvement	May be normal	CSF culture
Nocardia asteroïdes	1–6	Headache Localizing finding	Abscesses	Pleocytosis	Biopsy, CSF, blood culture
Aspergillus	1–6	Rapidly developing coma, seizures	Ring lesion, scattered hemorrhages	Pleocytosis	Biopsy, blood culture
Cryptococcus neoformans	>6	Unexplained headache, fever, cognitive changes, rarely focal signs	Thalamus, basal ganglia; widespread miliary	Pleocytosis; may be normal	CSF antigen
Toxoplasma gondii	>6	Seizures, stupor, rarely focal signs	Multiple lesions	Pleocytosis; may be normal	Brain biopsy, SPECT

CSF: cerebrospinal fluid; CT: computed tomography; IV: intravenously; MRI: magnetic resonance imaging; SPECT: single-photon emission computed tomography; TX: transplantation

Acute confusional state remains difficult to define in transplant recipients and can be considered if it lasts more than 2–3 consecutive days. Postoperative hyperactive delirium associated with hallucinations is common post transplantation, and some circumstances should be recognized.[7,9] Both hyperactive and hypoactive delirium after liver transplantation occurs in about a third of patients in the immediate postoperative period. This is seen more often in patients who had a pretransplant encephalopathy and in alcoholic liver disease. Often the hepatic encephalopathy is mild and self-limiting.

In a seriously confused patient there are many other causes that need to be considered. This includes, obviously, the use of calcineurin inhibitors, opioid antagonists, β-adrenergic blockers, and high-dose corticosteroids. All of these drugs can be implicated. Other commonly used drugs, such as midazolam and propofol, may impact level of consciousness, particularly because they have different pharmacokinetics in transplant patients. Midazolam, for example, although relatively short-acting in comparison with other sedative agents, has a prolonged activity if the liver graft is not functioning fully. It is also highly protein bound, and preexisting low protein levels may increase its sedative effects. Clearance of propofol is dependent on hepatic blood flow and cardiac output; if both are disturbed, awakening from propofol may be markedly delayed, and the patient may not awaken as usually anticipated 10–15 minutes after discontinuation of infusion. Opioids may continue to linger after cardiac transplantation; certainly when very large doses are used during the procedure.

In evaluating patients with impaired consciousness, some guidance can be provided. All potential sedative drugs should be looked at and the time remaining to clearance should be calculated. Physicians should consider administration of flumazenil or naloxone to eliminate the remaining effects.

One should obtain serum levels of cyclosporine or tacrolimus and trend the values. A marked increase in levels may indicate development of neurotoxicity, but such an association is only plausible if it is seen outside of the usual intravenous loading period (within the first week of treatment). Many transplant surgeons titrate toward increasing plasma levels—these levels should not be misinterpreted as indicative of neurotoxicity. Recent laboratory values should be obtained and should include electrolyte panel, liver and renal function tests, serum ammonia, arterial blood gas, and, where indicated, antiepileptic drug levels.[13,24] It is a mistake to label postoperative encephalopathy as multifactorial, if it means no effort will be made to find the possible triggers.

A liver transplant recipient may have severe hyponatremia, rising creatinine and BUN, and may show signs of early rejection; cefepime toxicity may be the cause of decline in consciousness and new myoclonus. Improvement is expected when the drug is discontinued.

The threshold for cerebrospinal fluid examination is low even if meningitis is not likely. Because an infectious mass lesion may be present, a CT scan may need to be performed to exclude such a lesion. In the case of an acutely febrile patient with an abnormal level of consciousness, an aggressive search for a CNS infection is recommended. These patients have a proclivity for infections with *Listeria monocytogenes*, *Nocardia*, and *Aspergillus*. Infections with *C. neoformans* or *T. gondii* are rarely seen within 6 months after transplantation.[31,34] All of these infections often show meningeal enhancement on a CT or MRI scan, solitary or multiple abscesses, or ring lesions. None of them are specific and the diagnosis can only be confirmed by biopsy, or occasionally by blood culture. The treatment is aggressive intravenous amphotericin, 1 mg/kg/day.

ORGAN TRANSPLANT–MORE SPECIFIC PROBLEMS

This chapter barely even scratches the surface of neurologic complications described over the years, but many are self-evident and predictable. The most common considerations are listed in Table 9.2 for easy reference.

Table 9.2 **Neurologic Signs in Transplant Recipients and Causes**

Sign	Causes
Failure to awaken	Hypoxic–ischemic brain injury (HX, LuX), Brain edema (LX), oversedation (LX), acute graft failure (LX, RX)
Acute Coma	Calcineurin neurotoxicity (LX), Intracranial hemorrhage (LX), Fulminant CNS infection (LX, HX)
Seizures	Calcineurin neurotoxicity (LX, RX), Intracranial hemorrhage (LX), Lymphoma (LX, HT, RX, LuX)
Aphasia, Dysarthria	Calcineurin neurotoxicity (LX, RX, LuX), Ischemic stroke (HX)
Hemiparesis	Brachial plexopathy (LX), Ischemic or hemorrhagic stroke, Brain tumor, Brain abscess (LX, HT, RX, LuX)
Tremors	Calcineurin neurotoxicity (LX, RX, LuX),
Myoclonus, Asterixis	Acute liver, renal, or pulmonary disease (LX, HT, RX, LuX), drug toxicity
Generalized weakness	Acute critical illness polyneuropathy, corticosteroid associated myopathy, neuromuscular blocking agents (LX, HT, RX, LuX)

HX: Heart transplant; LX: Liver transplant; LuX: Lung transplant; RX: Renal transplant

Lung transplant patients can face significant challenges in oxygenation and severe neurologic complications increases mortality. The most severe complications are perioperative stroke and encephalopathy. Acute hyperammonemia—an unexpected and not completely explained metabolic derangement in lung transplant recipients—has also been described; it causes seizures and profound encephalopathy.[18,19,29] Cyclosporin neurotoxicity is not a major cause of complications in lung transplant recipients.

Cardiac transplantations are obviously at risk of ischemic injury as a result of embolization from not only aortic atheroembolism but also perioperative cardiogenic shock, requiring extreme measures such as intraaortic balloon pump support or extracorporeal membrane oxygenation (ECMO). Intracerebral hemorrhage is rarely seen after cardiac transplantation, but poorly controlled hypertension may cause a lobar or basal ganglia hemorrhage.[30]

One relatively uncommon clinical scenario—at least in the United States—is a patient with acute fulminant hepatic failure followed by rapid listing for liver transplantation. This condition is unique, with many clinical uncertainties, and neurologists and neurosurgeons are often asked to be part of rapidly changing clinical decision-making process. Fulminant hepatic failure is a medical emergency, and liver transplantation is often the only effective treatment. Fulminant hepatic failure damages the brain, and thus the neurologist becomes involved.[5]

There are three immediate concerns. First, the transition of hepatic encephalopathy (basically a metabolic injury) to brain edema (now a structural injury)

must be recognized.[35] Second, intracranial pressure (ICP) may rise steeply and requires prompt treatment. Third, some patients may have already progressed to brain death, which would preclude transplantation. There have been multiple methods to identify patients with fulminant hepatic failure who might benefit from liver transplantation or who could be managed medically. Prognosis criteria proposed by Clichy are when hepatic encephalopathy is associated with a factor V concentration less than 20% if the patient is less than 30 years old (or less than 30% for those older than 30 years).[2] Age more than 50 years, time of jaundice to encephalopathy greater than 7 days, grade 3 to 4 hepatic encephalopathy, documented cerebral edema, prothrombin time more than 35 seconds, and serum creatinine more than 1.5 mg/dL may also be important deciding factors in a decision to proceed with liver transplantation. Poor prognosis is expected if any three of these factors are present. Other examples are the King's College Criteria and the MELD score. However, these prognostic factors have been criticized and in many instances found to be insufficient.[36]

Hepatic encephalopathy transitions to brain edema in untreated fulminant hepatic encephalopathy. The mechanism of brain edema in a fulminant hepatic failure is influenced by multiple factors. Hyperosmolarity is due to increased ammonia, but the development of oxidative stress may also contribute. Brain edema needs aggressive treatment, which is best guided with use of an ICP monitor.

Utilization of ICP monitors varies significantly between centers, with placement in approximately a quarter of the total patients seen with acute liver failure. Some centers use microdialysis to guide treatment.[14,17] The placement of an ICP device into the brain parenchyma has been concerning due to the associated coagulopathy. Data on the risks of ICP monitoring compiled from eight centers with experience in management of fulminant hepatic failure found intracranial hemorrhages in 10% of patients, including in patients who received fresh frozen plasma to control the coagulopathy.

Patients who receive ICP monitoring and are treated aggressively do not have a better outcome or higher percentage of liver transplantation and one could question the role of ICP-based management. Nonetheless, most centers proceed with insertion of an intraparenchymal ICP. Use of recombinant factor VII or prothrombin complex concentrate (PCC) are important new developments in countering coagulopathy in fulminant hepatic failure, and their use has significantly decreased the frequency of bleeding complications (during insertion of ICP device and the days thereafter). The optimal dose of recombinant factor VII is yet to be determined, but several studies have found that coagulopathy can be reversed with a low dose (5 μg/kg). The duration of the response to administration of factor VII is approximately 12 hours with the highest dose of 80 μg/kg. PCC may be equally effective. Close international normalized ratio (INR) and platelet monitoring is paramount.[27]

The mainstay of treatment of brain edema is osmotic therapy (mannitol or hypertonic saline). Hypertonic saline (3% or 23%) is also useful in patients who have developed hyponatremia. Cerebral blood flow can be controlled with hyperventilation and fluid removal with renal replacement therapy, and there has been interest in the use of indomethacin for uncontrolled surges in ICP.[8]

Hypothermia is an additional option. Experimental work has shown that mild hypothermia not only improves survival but also attenuates liver injury. Barbiturates may control ICP, but neurologic examination becomes unreliable for several days. Loss of brainstem reflexes should not be attributed to drug effects, and when CT scan shows brain edema (obliterated sulci and basal cisterns), a cerebral angiogram may be needed to document presence or absence of intracranial flow.

Intestinal transplantation for a short bowel syndrome due to thrombosis, inflammatory bowel disease, or radiation enteritis has become another "organ" transplantation, but experience is only in a few hundred patients.[37] The initial experience is not sufficient to potentially identify specific complications; most reported complications are in known categories such as encephalopathy, CNS infection, seizures, stroke, and neuromuscular complications. Early assessment suggests the rate of neurologic complications is much higher than in solid organ transplants.[1,15] In one series of 54 patients, three patients developed fatal cerebral aspergillosis,[36] and there were 11 instances of tacrolimus neurotoxicity. One possible explanation is the higher immunosuppression as a result of relative lower resistance to rejection of the intestine.[36]

Patients who have received hematopoietic cell transplantation do not, strictly speaking, fall under the heading of organ transplantation, but are worth discussing as a specific group that is more difficult to marshall.[4,25,30] The neurologic complications occur during harvesting and conditioning regimens and during the period of bone marrow aplasia and can occur after bone marrow reconstitution. Each of these procedures and events has specific complications, shown in Table 9.3.

Table 9.3 **Hematopoietic Cell Transplantation Complications**

Phase	Complications
Progenitor harvest and conditioning	• Drug toxicity Busulfan* Ifosfamide** Cytarabine*** Methotrexate****
Bone marrow aplasia	• Septic embolism (*Aspergillus* common) • Calcineurin inhibitor neurotoxicity • Bleeding
Bone marrow reconstitution	• Graft versus host disease[†] • Septic embolism (*toxoplasma* common)
Relapse of hematologic disorder	• Leukemic meningitis • Lymphoproliferative disorder

*seizures; **encephalopathy; ***cerebellar syndrome; ****myeloradiculopathy; †GBS-like picture, myopathy, muscle cramps

---

By the Way

- Neurologic complications after organ transplantation are declining
- Neurotoxicity from immunosuppressive agents remains prevalent
- Seizures are a common presentation of neurotoxicity
- Cerebral hematoma is seen with bone marrow and liver transplantation and is almost always fatal or markedly disabling
- Of all infections, fungal infections in transplant patients are the most worrisome and may progress to systemic fungemia

---

Neurologic Complications of Organ Recipients by the Numbers

- ~80% of cardiac transplant have a transient neurologic complication
- ~20% of transplants with a lymphoproliferative disorder have brain lesions
- ~5% of transplant patients may develop peripheral neuropathy
- ~3% of patients develop mononeuropathy or polyneuropathy
- ~2% of all transplant recipients may develop a neurologic infection
- ~1% of liver or cardiac transplants develop seizures

Putting It All Together

- There are perioperative risks leading to marked changes in oxygenation and blood pressure—all providing a constant challenge for the patient
- Abnormal pharmacokinetics may change drug clearance and increase the risk of abnormal consciousness
- CNS infections can be grouped in 6-month time periods; each has specific risks for certain organisms
- The management of fulminant hepatic failure leading to liver transplantation is complex, and patients may need close ICP control
- Hematopoietic cell transplantation recipients have a high proclivity to drug neurotoxicity causing seizures or cerebellar syndrome

References

1. Abu-Elmagd K, Reyes J, Bond G, et al. Clinical intestinal transplantation: a decade of experience at a single center. *Ann Surg* 2001;234:404–416.
2. Amodio P, Biancardi A, Montagnese S, et al. Neurological complications after orthotopic liver transplantation. *Dig Liver Dis* 2007;39:740–747.

3. Andrews BT, Hershon JJ, Calanchini P, et al. Neurologic complications of cardiac transplantation. *West J Med* 1990;153:146–148.

4. Antonini G, Ceschin V, Morino S, et al. Early neurologic complications following allogenic bone marrow transplant for leukemia: A prospective study. *Neurology* 1998;50:1441–1445.

5. Bernuau J, Goudeau A, Poynard T, et al. Multivariate analysis of prognostic factors in fulminant hepatitis B. *Hepatology* 1986;6:648–651.

6. Bronster DJ, Emre S, Boccagni P, et al. Central nervous system complications in liver transplant recipients—incidence, timing, and long-term follow up. *Clin Transplantation* 2000;14:1–7.

7. Buis CI, Wiesner RH, Krom RA, Kremers WK, Wijdicks EFM. Acute confusional state following liver transplantation for alcoholic liver disease. *Neurology* 2002;59:601–605.

8. Casey MJ, Meier-Kriesche HU. Calcineurin inhibitors in kidney transplantation: friend or foe? *Curr Opin Nephrol Hypertens* 2011;20:610–615.

9. Dhar R, Young GB, Marotta P. Perioperative neurological complications after liver transplantation are best predicted by pre-transplant hepatic encephalopathy. *Neurocrit Care* 2008;8:253–258.

10. Delios AM, Rosenblum M, Jakubowski AA, et al. Central and peripheral nervous system immune mediated demyelinating disease after allogeneic hemopoietic stem cell transplantation for hematologic disease. *J Neurooncol.* 2012;110:251–256.

11. Goldstein LS, Haug MT, Perl J, et al. Central nervous system complications after lung transplantation. *J Heart Lung Transplant* 1988;17:185–191.

12. Guarino M, Benito-Leon J, Decruyenaere J, et al. EFNS guidelines on management of neurological problems in liver transplantation. *Eur J Neurol* 2006;13:2–9.

13. Hocker S, Rabinstein AA, Wijdicks EFM. Pearls & oysters: status epilepticus from hyperammonemia after lung transplant. *Neurology* 2011;77:e54–e56.

14. Hutchinson PJ, Gimson A, Al-Rawi PG, et al. Microdialysis in the management of hepatic encephalopathy. *Neurocrit Care* 2006;5:202–205.

15. Idoate MA, Martinez AJ, Bueno J, Abu-Elmagd K, Reyes J. The neuropathology of intestinal failure and small bowel transplantation. *Acta Neuropathol* 1999;97:502–508.

16. Kamdar KY, Rooney CM, Heslop HE. Posttransplant lymphoproliferative disease following liver transplantation. *Curr Opin Organ Transplant* 2011;16:274–280.

17. Larsen FS. Is it worthwhile to use cerebral microdialysis in patients with acute liver failure? *Neurocrit Care* 2006;5:173–175.

18. Lyu DM, Zamora MR. Medical complications of lung transplantation. *Proc Am Thorac Soc* 2009;6:101–107.

19. Mateen FJ, Dierkhising RA, Rabinstein AA, van de Beek D, Wijdicks EFM. Neurological complications following adult lung transplantation. *Am J Transplant* 2010;10:908–914.

20. Mateen FJ, Muralidharan R, Carone M, et al. Progressive multifocal leukoencephalopathy in transplant recipients. *Ann Neurol* 2011;70:305–322.

21. Muñoz P, Valerio M, Palomo J, et al. Infectious and non-infectious neurologic complications in heart transplant recipients. *Medicine (Baltimore)* 2010;89:166–175.

22. O'Grady JG. Prognostication in acute liver failure: a tool or an anchor? *Liver Transpl* 2007;13:786–787.

23. Ranjan P, Mishra AM, Kale R, et al. Cytotoxic edema is responsible for raised intracranial pressure in fulminant hepatic failure: in vivo demonstration using diffusion-weighted MRI in human subjects. *Metab Brain Dis* 2005;20:181–192.

24. Rueda JF, Caldwell C, Brennan DC. Successful treatment of hyperammonemia after lung transplantation. *Ann Intern Med* 1998;128:956–957.

25. Saiz A, Graus F. Neurologic complications of hematopoietic cell transplantation. *Semin Neurol* 2010;30:287–295.

26. Saner FH, Sotiropoulos GC, Gu Y, et al. Severe neurological events following liver transplantation. *Arch Med Res* 2007;38:75–79.

27. Shami VM, Caldwell SH, Hespenheide EE, et al. Recombinant activated factor VII for coagulopathy in fulminant hepatic failure compared with conventional therapy. *Liver Transpl* 2003;9:138–143.

28. Shigemura N, Sclabassi RJ, Bhama JK, et al. Early major neurologic complications after lung transplantation: incidence, risk factors, and outcome. *Transplantation*. 2103;95:866–871.

29. Taylor AL, Watson CJ, Bradley JA. Immunosuppressive agents in solid organ transplantation: mechanisms of action and therapeutic efficacy. *Crit Rev Oncol Hematol* 2005;56:23–46.

30. Van de Beek D, Kremers W, Daly RC, et al. Effect of neurologic complications on outcome after heart transplant. *Arch Neurol* 2008;65:226–231.

31. Van de Beek D, Patel R, Daly RC, et al. Central nervous system infections in heart transplant recipients. *Arch Neurol* 2007;64:1715–1720.

32. Vaquero J, Belanger M, James L, et al. Mild hypothermia attenuates liver injury and improves survival in mice with acetaminophen toxicity. *Gastroenterology* 2007;132:372–383.

33. Wijdicks EFM, Plevak DJ, Wiesner RH, Steers JL. Causes and outcome of seizures in liver transplant recipients. *Neurology* 1996;47:1523–1525.

34. Wijdicks EFM (ed.). *Neurologic Complications in Organ Transplant Recipients*. Boston, Butterworth-Heinemann, 1999.

35. Wijdicks EFM. Impaired consciousness after liver transplantation. *Liver Transpl Surg.* 1995;1:329–334.

36. Yantorno SE, Kremers WK, Ruf AE, et al. MELD is superior to King's College and Clichy's criteria to assess prognosis in fulminant hepatic failure. *Liver Transpl* 2007;13:822–828.

37. Zivković SA, Eidelman BH, Bond G, Costa G, Abu-Elmagd KM. The clinical spectrum of neurologic disorders after intestinal and multivisceral transplantation. *Clin Transplant* 2010;24:164–168.

10

Troubleshooting: Easily Overlooked CT Scan Signs

The surest and quickest way to find a cause for acute brain injury is a CT scan of the brain and is available in medical centers admitting acutely ill patients. Even with the rapid availability of MR imaging in tertiary care centers throughout the world, a CT scan of the brain remains the most frequently utilized imaging modality. In most instances decisions are initially based on a "plain" CT scan of the brain, and CT angiogram, CT venogram, or CT perfusion scans are performed with critical indications. CT scan of the brain is usually obtained in a radiology suite, but portable CT scans are available. Exposure to ionizing radiation may become a concern if the study can be obtained too easily.

Once the image is done, careful assessment of it is a major responsibility of the neurologist, who cannot afford to simply read a final report—as so many other physicians do. It therefore would seem like a truism that any neurologist should view a CT scan himself.[8] In reality, CT scans in major hospitals are seen by radiologists and often neuroradiologists; but after hours and at night the interpretation is provided by residents in training.[17,29] Emergency physicians are also judging the findings on noncontrast CT scans of the brain, but when their interpretation is audited, they are only correct about two-thirds of the time.[14,33] Teleradiology may change the entire picture—literally.

In some countries there continues to be debate about the true need for a CT scan beyond working hours or even working days.[28] This discussion involves the need for CT of the brain in trauma (Chapter 3). It has been argued that the availability of a CT scan may increase its use and paradoxically delay treatment. For example, one canadian study found that a CT scan before a lumbar puncture resulted in a door-to-antibiotic time of 6 hours in patients with bacterial meningitis.[24] In the UK, scoring systems have been created to identify patients who have a high proclivity for intracranial hemorrhage after presenting with "stroke symptoms" and, conversely, to defer CT scans if the probability of hemorrhage is low—a situation that would be quite problematic in the litigious atmosphere of the United States.[23] It would be very unusual—and perhaps even substandard care—in the United States for any patient with transient or persistent neurologic symptoms that potentially could indicate a recent brain lesion not to undergo a CT scan.

There is another concern. There may be a disconnect between CT scan findings and clinical diagnosis and substantial clinical experience is required to sort this out. This can be illustrated by two examples. Cerebral abscess in a febrile patient may show a vague hypodensity on plain CT scan but a ring-enhancing lesion after contrast. A cerebral venous thrombosis may have a virtually normal CT scan only to become clear after CT venogram (CTV) studies. CT scan can be normal in early meningitis, encephalitis, anoxic-ischemic injury, and even in traumatic brain injury. In severely affected patients, however, CT later becomes abnormal or MRI may have already demonstrated the abnormalities sought for.

Extensive experience over the years has resulted in the recognition of patterns of errors perhaps best summarized as "the overlooked CT scan." Of course, the abnormalities are all subtle, but consequences are not necessarily minor. Missing a hyperdense middle cerebral artery (MCA) or basilar artery sign may not lead to endovascular intervention, a missed subarachnoid hemorrhage (SAH) may not lead to cerebrospinal fluid (CSF) examination or cerebral angiogram and a missed string sign may not lead to a CTV or MR venogram (MRV).

Where do we go wrong, and how can we recognize these misjudgments? This chapter presents some of these scenarios.

Basic Neuroradiological Skills

In order to understand how errors are made, normal anatomy of the brain on CT scan should be known. There are a plethora of normal variants, some of which can lead to misinterpretation.

The first order of business is to evaluate the CT scan for orientation and windows. The plane is usually parallel to the orbitomeatal line (from the eye to the external auditory meatus). However, the gantry might be seriously tilted, or the patient may have moved during scanning, which creates a different plane and can also lead to a failure to image key structures. This is particularly pertinent in the slices where the basal cisterns are imaged. In patients with SAH, this image fluke may be a cause of a false-negative CT scan. Significant asymmetries may lead to failure to image a nonaerated mastoid sinus from mastoiditis associated with fulminant bacterial meningitis. Abnormalities in the posterior fossa may also go undetected, such as in an evolving cerebral infarct.

The CT windows settings have a typical width. Hounsfield units (HU) are arbitrarily set at 0 for CSF and at –1,000 for air. Usually CT operates within 60–80 HU; this provides the best differentiation between gray and white matter (CSF is at 15 HU, blood is at 30–50 HU). Increasing this window to approximately 200 HU may better separate a small rim of hyperdensity, such as a subdural hematoma, from bone.

An HU window in the 2,000 range will best image bone structures and changes in this window change the gray scale. The CT be scrutinized for fractures and, as mentioned above, aeration of mastoids—they may be filled with blood or pus.

Most emergency CT scans are without intravenous contrast and difficult to obtain outside working hours. CT scans, however, may show contrast if a prior contrast examination of another structure has been performed, such as coronary angiogram for acute myocardial infarction, CT of the chest for pulmonary emboli, or CT of the abdomen for trauma. This may make assessment of cerebral hemorrhage or SAH very difficult, because blood and contrast have roughly similar HU (dual energy CT may differentiate between the two).

It is useful to start reading of the CT scan by systematically identifying structures below the tentorium and above the tentorium (Figure 10.1). These slices are usually reviewed from bottom to top. Below the tentorium, the medulla oblongata, cerebellar tonsils, and vertebral artery can often be identified in the foramen magnum. The vertebral artery is often hyperdense and may contain small calcifications. The presence of cerebellar tonsils has very little meaning, because they can be present in normal conditions. (Its presence—in certain brain injuries—is inaccurately used to be indicative of increased intracranial pressure). A higher cut will identify a the pons and cerebellar hemispheres. At this level, the bone window should be scrutinized for abnormalities of the mastoids and frontal sinuses. Specific attention to a possible hyperdense basilar artery is necessary, because CT scans can be normal despite the presence of an acute embolus—hypodensities in

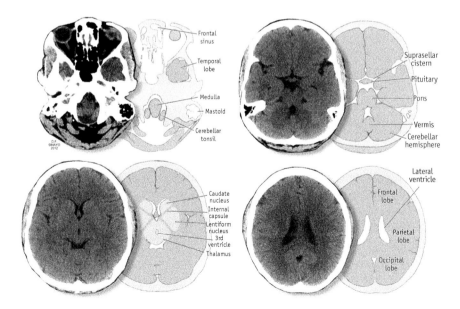

Figure 10.1 CT Scan Structures that should be identified.

the pons and cerebellum indicating infarction may take 12–24 hours to emerge on CT. The eye positioning could also show a forced-eye deviation that should be already known clinically. It is a common CT finding in acute hemispheric stroke. (not all patients with conjugate eye deviation have a major stroke—it may be simply a matter of the patient looking sideways during scanning).[27]

In a higher cut, the pentagonial structure of the basal cisterns is identified. These are located anterior to the midbrain, and the surrounding cisterns should be identified if the structure is not pentagonial but rounded off, which may indicate a mass (sometimes a pituitary tumor). The temporal horns of the ventricles are seen at this level, and when if prominent, they may be indicative of an obstructive hydrocephalus. CT slices further identify gray and white matter differentiation of the brain parenchyma, particularly in the lentiform nucleus, caudate, insular cortex, and internal capsule. The thalamus is identified close to the calcified pineal gland. In the highest cuts, the falx is identified, as is the body of the lateral ventricle.

Interpretation of CT scan of the brain should also specifically address the presence of blood. This appears hyperdense and may initially become more hyperdense, followed by isodensity. Density usually changes within the first week, and blood may have the same density as brain in approximately 3–4 weeks. This is particularly pertinent in patients with a subdural hematoma. Extradural hemorrhage has a biconvex configuration. A subdural hemorrhage has a crescent-shaped configuration. Subarachnoid hemorrhage is in cisterns, fissures, and sulci. Intracranial hemorrhages are typically located in either a lobe, putamen, caudate, or thalamus.

All cisterns and ventricles should be identified and, if not seen, may indicate compression from a lesion. One should identify the fourth, third, and lateral ventricles and whether there is obstructive hydrocephalus. An absent third ventricle might indicate a colloid cyst that has identical density as the brain and may be easily missed. Not seeing an identifiable fourth ventricle might indicate mass effect from a cerebellar lesion; its absence is important in judging the seriousness of the condition.

The parenchyma is again clearly scrutinized for the presence of calcifications, hypodense and hyperdense regions, and also changes in gray-white differentiation. Abnormalities and disappearance of the gray-white differentiation in the caudate and the lentiform nucleus can occur within hours of presentation of an ischemic stroke. The cortical sulci should be identified, left and right, and it should be noted whether there are assymetries. One can expect less prominent sulci in young individuals, and as a reflection of normal aging more prominent sulci in older patients. A CT scan that does not fit the age, also known as a "hypernormal CT scan," may point to bilateral isodense subdural hematomas.

Finally, the bone sections are again reviewed. Cortical bone fractures or tumors (with erosion) should be looked for. Sometimes the abnormality is on the very last cut.

Identifying the Problem

This chapter cannot list all subtleties, but Table 10.1 shows the most commonly missed abnormalities on brain CT and many have been published. A series of CT scans is shown (but without arrows to replicate real situations and to challenge the reader a bit). A common problem is the failure to recognize new blood from SAH. Some examples are shown in Figure 10.2. Aneurysmal SAH is typically easily recognized finding blood in basal cisterns, fissures, and sulci. Inappropriate imaging that results in failure to visualize the basal cisterns may be a cause of missed SAH. Blood can be subtle, present in the posterior horns of the ventricles, sylvian fissure, or prepontine region—sometimes a tiny clot of a few pixels may be seen in the interpeduncular cistern. A small hemorrhage in front of the pons may also be a retroclival hematoma. There is a great likelihood that the history will reveal a significant trauma and follow-up studies should look for cervical spine luxations or odontoid fracture.[7]

The sensitivity of a CT scan for SAH is quite high. A recent study that included all patients with acute headache—but likely a small proportion of thunderclap headaches—found 240 of 3,132 (7.7%) had a negative CT and SAH confirmed only by lumbar puncture. The sensitivity of CT scanning was nearly 100% in the first 6 hours, though with a 3% possibility of missing an SAH. The sensitivity did decrease substantially if patients were seen more than 6 hours after presentation.[23] Whether finding this will lead to reduced lumbar punctures is unclear, and the practice of a CT scan followed by lumbar puncture continues to be important if patients present with a headache that is unexpected and unusually severe.

False positive SAH may appear on CT scans in patients (after prolonged cardiopulmonary resuscitation). Loss of gray-white differentiation, loss of sulci, and appearance of vascular structures (arteries and veins) rather than diffuse blood clots clinches the diagnosis. (Clinically it may still be difficult to separate the two, since SAH may present with cardiac arrest.)[32] This finding on CT is very often

Table 10.1 **CT Scans with Overlooked or Misinterpreted Signs**

- Subarachnoid hemorrhage (overlooked or not imaged)
- Occipital infarcts (overlooked)
- Skull fractures (overlooked or not imaged)
- Mass in sella (overlooked)
- Hyperdense middle cerebral artery or basilar artery sign (overlooked)
- Tumor (interpreted as stroke)
- Posterior reversible encephalopathy syndrome (interpreted as stroke)
- Cerebral venous thrombosis (interpreted as spontaneous cerebral hemorrhage)

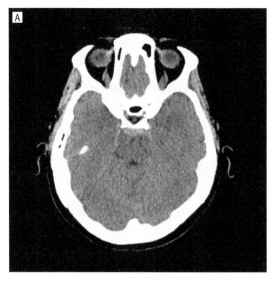

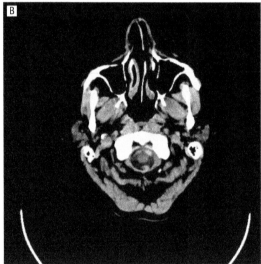

Figure 10.2 CT examples of subtle subarachnoid blood. A: prepontine;
B: cervicomedullary junction.

misinterpreted as SAH and may even become the final diagnosis on a death cer-
tificate (Figure 10.3).

Another commonly missed feature on CT scan is a hyperdense MCA rep-
resenting clot (Figure 10.4). A false negative hyperdense MCA sign may be a
streak-like hemorrhage that may turn out to be a ruptured MCA aneurysm.

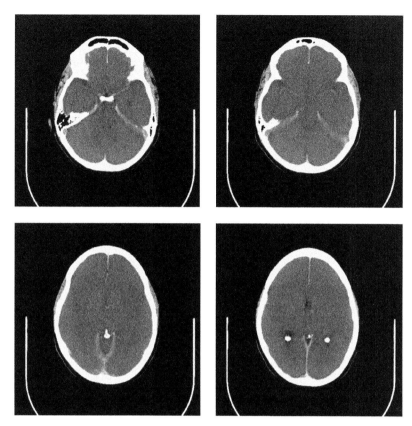

Figure 10.3 Pseudo subarachnoid hemorrhage. Note loss of gray-white differentiation and loss of sulci.

A false positive hyperdense MCA sign may be seen in patients with a temporal lobe hypodensity—we have seen that repeatedly with herpes simplex encephalitis.[19] Other common false-positive hyperdense MCA signs are due to calcinosis, high hematocrit, or tumor causing a hypodensity of the temporal lobe and relative hyperdensity of the MCA branch. HU measurement of the hyperdense MCA sign may be helpful but is far from accurate; however, the chances of a pseudo hyperdense MCA sign are greater with HU above 43.[13,15]

Perhaps the most commonly missed abnormality in acute stroke is a hyperdense basilar artery sign. There are several reasons for this. The disorder is uncommon and not clinically considered even if there are clinical pointers such as acute coma with anisocoria and thus extensor posturing. The basilar artery is always "somewhat" hyperdense and not recognized as abnormal (Figure 10.5). CT streak artifacts and common occurrence of atherosclerosis in the posterior circulation reduce the accuracy of a hyperdense basilar artery sign. Moreover,

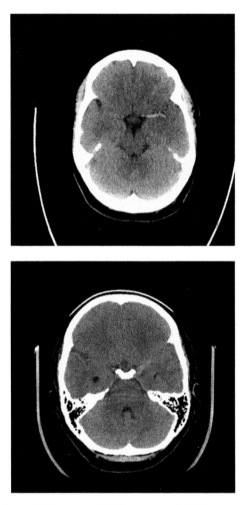

Figure 10.4 Hyperdense MCA sign and "false positive" (SAH misread as MCA hyperdensity).

there is no paired artery for comparison as there is in the anterior circulation. Again, when HU is used as a cutoff value for true positives and false positives, an HU of 40–42 only has a sensitivity of 78%, specificity of 83%, and accuracy of 80%.[6] If a positive hyperdense basilar artery sign is further imaged with MRA, one study found only 9 of 61 "positive hyperdense basilar artery signs with true embolus."[30] In the appropriate clinical setting a hyperdense basilar artery sign indicating a basilar artery embolus should immediately lead to a CTA or MRA.

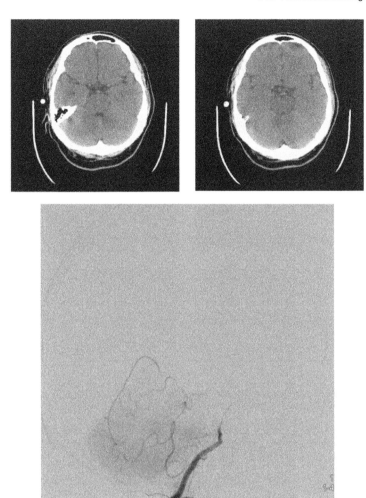

Figure 10.5 Hyperdense basilar artery sign on CT scan, confirmed basilar artery thrombus on cerebral angiogram.

A common misinterpretation is not recognizing the early signs of cerebral infarction. Early effacement of caudate and putamen and loss of the cortical ribbon may not be recognized and may require changing the windows. The early signs of ischemia with loss of the insular ribbon and lentiform nucleus (Figure 10.6) are already noted within the first hours. In major territory ischemia, parenchymal hypodensity may appear with 6 hours, and sulcal effacement within 12 hours; but there is a significant variation in appearance, and exact timing is not possible.[26] Another common misinterpretation is diagnosing an ischemic stroke while a tumor is present. In the past, before MRI scan, such misinterpretation led to

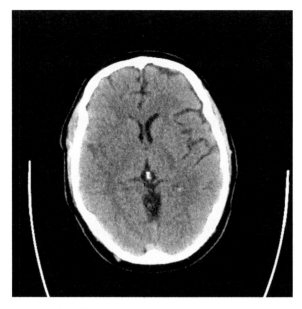

Figure 10.6 Loss of insular ribbon, lentiform nucleus, and cortical definition.

inappropriate biopsies and even explorations and decompressive craniotomies. Usually the hypodensity is outside a vascular territory, and the findings on examination are minimal.

It would seem counterintuitive that errors can be made with an intracerebral hemorrhage, because the abnormality is hard to miss. One study suggested that a combination of clinical information and neuroradiological information, using the so-called SCAN rule (4 predictor variables—S, severe hypertension at onset; C, confusion at onset; A, prior anticoagulation; N, nausea or vomiting at onset) increased the likelihood of intracranial hemorrhage being identified on CT scan.[18]

It is important to remember that not every intracranial hemorrhage is arterial.[16] Cerebral venous thrombosis on CT scan should be considered in any patient with an intracranial hemorrhage in the temporal or occipital lobe, or hemorrhagic conversion of an ischemic stroke. A string sign or hyperintensity in the falx should be specifically looked for and has immediate consequences for ordering of the next test, either a MRV or CTV (Figure 10.7). Some hemorrhages are a hemorrhagic conversion of an infarct, and some are hemorrhages associated with infection or underlying vascular lesions. Finally with interpretation of intracranial hemorrhages, neurologists should be aware that one of the major pitfalls is hemorrhage into the temporal lobe from herpes simplex encephalitis and that leads to a completely different treatment.

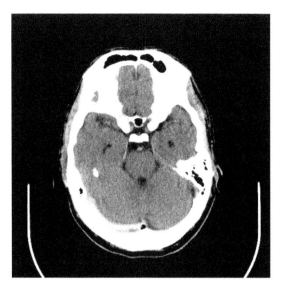

Figure 10.7 String sign (close to occiput) in cerebral venous thrombosis.

Most lobar hematomas are without an underlying structural lesion, but a cerebral angiogram or CTA may be needed. This is clearly illustrated in Figure 10.8, where a CT showed a somewhat surprising MCA aneurysm in a lobar hematoma without appreciable SAH. Conversely, intracerebral hemorrhage may also be misdiagnosed in small hyperdense lesions due to cavernous malformations (Figure 10.9) or when a calcification is present (Figure 10.10).

Incidental findings are also common on MRI. Most have no consequences, and many may not be mentioned. Examples are lacunar infarcts or sulci misinterpreted as infarction. When 2,000 MRIs were studied in normal volunteers, lacunar infarcts were found in 6%, cerebral infarction in 7%, aneurysm in 2%, benign brain tumor in 2%, arachnoid cyst in 1%, and a variety of other abnormalities in under 1%.[31]

Practical Issues

Most of the quality studies have involved examination of discrepancy rates between residents and staff, and between radiology residents and neuroradiology fellows, and also second-opinion consultations by staff in neuroradiology with overnight evaluations.[33] Overall discrepancy rates are not too bad and vary from 3% to 14%;[1,5,10,20,21] and the discrepancies that have been identified do not

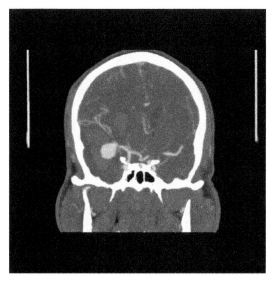

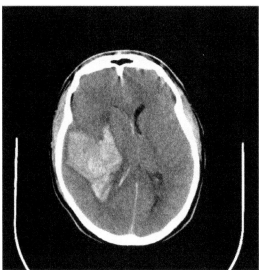

Figure 10.8 Lobar hematoma from MCA aneurysm.

always lead to change in management or a different outcome. One study found that on-call radiology residents had a 0.9% rate of significant misinterpretation, but only in 0.08% was there a potentially serious effect on patient outcome.[17,22] Quality control between fellowship-trained neuroradiologists on staff at a major academic medical center found a 2% rate of clinically significant detection of interpretation discrepancy. Generally, it is known that compared with community

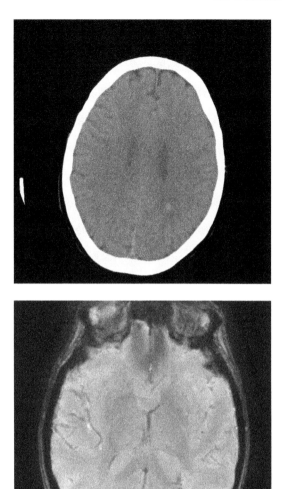

Figure 10.9 Venous angioma misread as ICH and confirmed on MRI.

hospitals, academic medical centers have error rates that are not much more than 1%.[3,4] Common misjudgments in emergency CT scans include subdural hematoma along the tentorium that was read as normal, pneumocephalus that was read as normal, acute hemorrhagic infarction that was interpreted as a calcified infarction, remote infarction interpreted as a postoperative change, and a misjudged skull fracture.[8] Missed findings included sellar or supersellar masses, a cerebellar

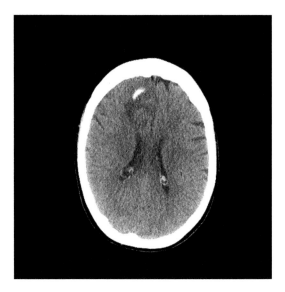

Figure 10.10 Calcification with oligodendroglioma misread as ICH.

mass, small hemorrhagic contusions, hyperdense MCA sign, subarachnoid hemorrhage after trauma, a subdural hematoma in an infant, and an acute blowout fracture.[10]

Overnight CT scan interpretations also missed intracranial hemorrhages, and the discrepancies were usually seen in subdural hemorrhage and SAH.[25] Missed subdural hematomas were mostly located frontally, parafalcine, and subtentorially. Most commonly overlooked contusions were in the temporal and frontal lobe. SAH included overlooked blood in the interpeduncular cisterns, sylvian fissure, and diffusely localized blood in the cortex. The most common patterns that were incorrectly identified were a hemorrhagic contusion, epidural hematoma, or a shear injury from a head injury.[21]

Finally, another common problem during overnight CT scanning is the absence of administration of contrast. Occasional cases are published that show a CT scan with a hypodensity that after contrast demonstrates a ring-enhancing lesion that could be a bacterial abscess or metastasis.[2]

Putting It All Together

- CT scans done early after onset of acute brain injury may not identify important pathology
- CT scan sensitivity for ICH and SAH (within 6 hours) is very high.
- Most commonly missed abnormalities are due to failure to obtain CTA or CTV

- Hyperdensity (meaning visible clot) in large cerebral arteries is not always recognized
- Early signs of cerebral ischemia are loss of putamen and caudate structures with loss of the cortical ribbon surrounding these structures
- Most CT errors come during the night hours and include failure to recognize contusions and subdural hematomas

References

1. Alfaro D, Levitt MA, English DK, Williams V, Eisenberg R. Accuracy of interpretation of cranial computed tomography scans in an emergency medicine residency program. *Ann Emerg Med* 1995;25:169–174.
2. Bagga V, Simons MA. Cerebral abscesses—a stroke mimic. *Age Ageing* 2011;40:645.
3. Borgstede JP, Lewis RS, Bhargavan M, Sunshine JH. RADPEER quality assurance program: a multifacility study of interpretive disagreement rates. *J Am Coll Radiol* 2004;1:59–65.
4. Bossuyt PM, Reitsma JB, Bruns DE, et al. Towards complete and accurate reporting of studies of diagnostic accuracy: the STARD initiative. *AJR Am J Roentgenol.* 2003;181:51–55.
5. Bruni SG, Bartlett E, Yu E. Factors involved in discrepant preliminary radiology resident interpretations of neuroradiological imaging studies: a retrospective analysis. *AJR Am J Roentgenol* 2012;198:1367–1374.
6. Connell L, Koerte IK, Laubender RP, et al. Hyperdense basilar artery sign: a reliable sign of basilar artery occlusion. *Neuroradiology* 2012;54:321–327.
7. Datar S, Daniel S, Wijdicks EFM. A major pitfall to avoid: retroclival hematoma due to odontoid fracture: *Neurocrit Care* 2013;19:206–209.
8. Erly WK, Ashdown BC, Lucio RW 2nd, et al. Evaluation of emergency CT scans of the head: is there a community standard? *AJR Am J Roentgenol* 2003;180:1727–1730.
9. Erly WK, Berger WG, Krupinski E, Seeger JF, Guisto JA. Radiology resident evaluation of head CT scan orders in the emergency department. *AJNR Am J Neuroradiol* 2002;23:103–107.
10. Filippi CG, Schneider B, Burbank HN, et al. Discrepancy rates of radiology resident interpretations of on-call neuroradiology MR imaging studies. *Radiology* 2008;249:972–979.
11. Grotta JC, Chiu D, Lu M, et al. Agreement and variability in the interpretation of early CT changes in stroke patients qualifying for intravenous rtPA therapy. *Stroke* 1999;30:1528–1533.
12. Heckmann JG. A note on the hyperdense middle cerebral artery sign. *Emerg Med J* 2013;30:345
13. Jha B, Kothari M. Pearls & oysters: hyperdense or pseudohyperdense MCA sign: a Damocles sword? *Neurology* 2009;72:e116–e117.
14. Khoo NC, Duffy M. Out of hours non-contrast head CT scan interpretation by senior emergency department medical staff. *Emerg Med Australas* 2007;19:122–128.
15. Koo CK, Teasdale E, Muir KW. What constitutes a true hyperdense middle cerebral artery sign? *Cerebrovasc Dis* 2000;10:419–423.
16. Krasnokutsky MV. Cerebral venous thrombosis: a potential mimic of primary traumatic brain injury in infants. *AJR Am J Roentgenol* 2011;197:W503–W507.
17. Lal NR, Murray UM, Eldevik OP, Desmond JS. Clinical consequences of misinterpretations of neuroradiologic CT scans by on-call radiology residents. *AJNR Am J Neuroradiol* 2000;21:124–129.
18. Lovelock CE, Redgrave JN, Briley D, Rothwell PM. The SCAN rule: a clinical rule to reduce CT misdiagnosis of intracerebral hemorrhage in minor stroke. *J Neurol Neurosurg Psychiatry* 2010;81:271–275.

19. Maramattom BV, Wijdicks EFM. A misleading hyperdense MCA sign. *Neurology* 2004;63:586.
20. Miyakoshi A, Nguyen QT, Cohen WA, Talner LB, Anzai Y. Accuracy of preliminary interpretation of neurologic CT examinations by on-call radiology residents and assessment of patient outcomes at a level I trauma center. *J Am Coll Radiol* 2009;6:864–870.
21. Mucci B, Brett C, Huntley LS, Greene MK. Cranial computed tomography in trauma: the accuracy of interpretation by staff in the emergency department. *Emerg Med J* 2005;22:538–540.
22. Mukerji N, Cahill J, Paluzzi A, et al. Emergency head CT scans: can neurosurgical registrars be relied upon to interpret them? *Br J Neurosurg* 2009;23:158–161.
23. Perry JJ, Stiell IG, Sivilotti ML, et al. Sensitivity of computed tomography performed within six hours of onset of headache for diagnosis of subarachnoid hemorrhage: prospective cohort study. *BMJ* 2011;343:d4277.
24. Proulx N, Fréchette D, Toye B, Chan J, Kravcik S. Delays in the administration of antibiotics are associated with mortality from adult acute bacterial meningitis. *QJM* 2005;98:291–298.
25. Ravindran V, Sennik D, Hughes RA. Appropriateness of out-of-hours CT head scans. *Emerg Radiol* 2007;13:181–185.
26. Sarikaya B, Provenzale J. Frequency of various brain parenchymal findings of early cerebral ischemia on unenhanced CT scans. *Emerg Radiol* 2010;17:381–390.
27. Schwartz KM, Ahmed AT, Fugate JE, et al. Frequency of eye deviation in stroke and non-stroke patients undergoing head CT. *Neurocrit Care* 2012;17:45–48.
28. Stiell IG, Clement CM, Rowe BH, et al. Comparison of the Canadian CT Head Rule and the New Orleans Criteria in patients with minor head injury. *JAMA* 2005;294:1511–1518.
29. Strub WM, Leach JL, Tomsick T, Vagal A. Overnight preliminary head CT interpretations provided by residents: locations of misidentified intracranial hemorrhage. *AJNR Am J Neuroradiol* 2007;28:1679–1682.
30. Tan X, Guo Y. Hyperdense basilar artery sign diagnoses acute posterior circulation stroke and predicts short-term outcome. *Neuroradiology* 2010;52:1071–1078.
31. Vernooij MW et al. Incidental findings on brain MRI in the general population. *N Eng J Med* 2007;357:1821–1828.
32. Wong LC, Schelvan C, Mitchell LA, Inwald DP. Computed tomography may demonstrate pseudosubarachnoid hemorrhage in diffuse cerebral edema after cardiorespiratory arrest. *Pediatr Crit Care Med* 2011;12:e208–e210.
33. Yaniv G, Mozes O, Greenberg G, et al. Common sites and etiologies of residents' misinterpretation of head CT scans in the emergency department of a level I trauma center. *Isr Med Assoc J* 2013;15:221–225.
34. Zan E, Yousem DM, Carone M, Lewin JS. Second-opinion consultations in neuroradiology. *Radiology* 2010;255:135–141.

Index

brainstem
  coma 2, 4–6, 8
  encephalitis 64
  mass effect 72, 74
breath odor 9
breathing, respiratory failure 100–2, 102f, 108
bulbocavernosus reflex 48

calcification 142f
calcineurin inhibitors 117–19, 121
calcium 6, 19, 35
Canadian Head CT scan rule 36
cancer. See tumors
carbon dioxide, hypercapnia 101–2, 105–6, 108
cardiac arrhythmias 6, 14, 20
cardiac transplantation 116–17, 121, 122
cardiomyopathy 20
carotid artery occlusion 84, 90
CASPR2 autoantibodies 60, 61
catecholamines 20
cauda equina syndrome 47
caudate 132, 137
cefepime 121
ceftriaxone 12
central cord syndrome 47
cerebellum 2, 4, 74, 75–76, 131
cerebral edema 33, 73, 74, 117, 118, 123–24
cerebral hemorrhage
  after cardiac transplant 122
  imaging 132, 133–34, 134f, 138–39, 142
  surgery 71, 72–73, 74–77, 77f, 78
cerebrospinal fluid (CSF)
  in diagnosis 60, 62, 64, 121
  hydrocephalus 11, 74, 78, 132
cervical injury 39, 50–52, 51f
children
  encephalitis 64
  respiratory failure 106
  safeguarding 40
  TBI 36, 40
clinical examination
  in coma 7–10
  in spinal cord injury 47–49
clonazepam 21
coagulation profile, surgery and 39, 53, 79
coagulopathy 117, 123
coil embolization 75
coma 1–14
  diagnosis of cause 1–4, 7–10
  encephalitis 12, 65
  localization 4–6, 8
  management 6–7, 10–14
  TBI 2, 12, 33, 40
computed tomography (CT) 129–30
  angiograms 74–75, 91, 139
  anoxic–ischemic injury 133–34, 135f
  cerebral hematoma/hemorrhage 74–75, 132, 133–34, 134f, 139, 140f, 142
  coma 5, 10

contrast 86–88, 87f, 131, 142
infections 67, 120, 130, 135, 138
ischemic stroke 10, 85–88, 91, 131–32, 134–38, 136f, 137f, 138f
problems in interpretation 133–39
quality control 141–42
reading a scan 130–32, 131f
spinal cord injury 50
TBI 34f, 35–36, 38, 133
transplant patients 118, 120, 121
tumors 79, 137–38, 141f, 142f
venous thrombosis 130, 138, 139f
confusion 119–21
contactin-2 autoantibodies 60
contrast CT scans 86–88, 87f, 131, 142
contusions, cerebral 33–34, 34f, 40, 76
corticosteroids
  in autoimmune encephalitis 67
  in spinal cord injury 50, 54
  in status epilepticus 23
  to reduce ICP 11–12
cough 102, 105
Cryptococcus neoformans 120
crystalloids 6
CSF. See cerebrospinal fluid
CT. See computed tomography
cyclophosphamide 63, 67–68
cyclosporin 117–19, 121
cytomegalovirus 64, 65

death, in status epilepticus 25
decompressive craniectomy 12, 39–40, 74, 76–78, 77f
delirium 119–21
demyelination on EMG 103
deterioration 5–6, 33–35, 72, 75
dexamethasone 12, 54
diabetes 7, 12
diaphragm, in respiratory failure 100–2, 106
  functional tests 103–5, 104f
diazepam 21
diet, ketogenic 25
Duret hemorrhage 72–73
dyspnea. See respiratory failure
dystonia 60

electroencephalography (EEG)
  in coma 10
  in encephalitis 65
  in status epilepticus 19, 21, 25
electrolyte disturbances 9
electromyography (EMG) 103, 104f
embolism. See thromboembolism
embolization coils 75
encephalitis 59–69
  autoimmune 60–63, 62f, 66, 67–68
  imaging 12, 60, 65, 67, 120, 135, 138
  management 12, 62–63, 65–68
  viral 12, 63–65, 67, 119, 135, 138